AF379849

Uncemented Femoral Stems for Revision Surgery

Pierre Le Béguec · François Canovas
Olivier Roche · Mathias Goldschild · Julien Batard

Uncemented Femoral Stems for Revision Surgery

The Press-fit Concept - Planning - Surgical Technique - Evaluation

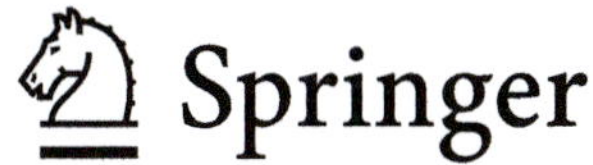

Pierre Le Béguec
Rennes
France

François Canovas
Hôpital Lapeyronie
Montpellier cedex
France

Olivier Roche
Centre Chirurgical Emile Gallé
Nancy
France

Mathias Goldschild
Polyclinique Sévigné
Cesson-Sévigné
France

Julien Batard
Hôpital Lapeyronie
Montpellier cedex
France

ISBN 978-3-319-03613-7   ISBN 978-3-319-03614-4   (eBook)
DOI 10.1007/978-3-319-03614-4
Springer Heidelberg New York Dordrecht London

Translation from the French language edition 'Reprise des prothèses fémorales descellées' © Sauramps Medical, Montpellier, 2013; ISBN: 9782840230625

Library of Congress Control Number: 2015934231

Printed on acid-free paper

Springer is part of Springer Science+Business Media (www.springer.com)

1. This monograph is not an exhaustive survey of the various femoral prostheses and surgical techniques available for the treatment of loosened femoral stems, namely revisions with cemented femoral stems will be not addressed in this study.
   This monograph discusses the revision of loosened femoral prostheses by means of an uncemented femoral stem system.
2. Ensuring reliable primary stability for an uncemented implant is achieved in different ways, depending on the chosen concept and the design of the implant.
   This book refers to uncemented, straight femoral stems whose primary stability is achieved by means of an intimate surface contact between bone and implant.
   It is also important to remember that it is not possible to use a straight and a curved stem in the same manner and the modularity is not a concept in itself to ensure primary stability of an uncemented femoral implant. The modularity is only a means efficient for the preparation of the anchorage zone and for the choice of the right implant.
3. Finally, it should be pointed out that this monograph was written fully independently; the authors were not biased in their work, especially not when assessing the results.

June 2013

Acknowledgments

The authors thank F. Bonnomet and J. Girard for their participation in the development of the evaluation method of the radiological results and the analysis of the results, as well as J.C. Murie for the drawings and A. Ingels for the statistical studies.

Contents

Part IV   Evaluation of Radiographic Results – How?

Preamble

First Part: Press-Fit Concept

In a first step, the surgeon has to select a concept to ensure primary stability of an uncemented implant, and to avoid serious errors, at the time of choosing a surgical strategy, it is necessary to acquire a perfect knowledge of the objectives imposed by the chosen concept.

The press-fit concept offers real guarantees to ensure the primary stability of an uncemented implant. Failures of this method are often due to an insufficient understanding of the prerequisites for this concept. Conversely, a surgeon who has a clear perception of the objectives that must be reached will make, always more easily, technical gestures that might, at first, appear not obvious or excessive.

"To explain a failure, often it is not the implant which is in question, but the way to use it"

Second Part: Preoperative Planning

The quality of a surgical gesture does not depend on the manual skills of the surgeon performing it, but on how he has prepared and performed the gesture "virtually", before actually performing it. There is a narrow correlation between the way of thinking about a surgical act and its implementation. This is accurately conveyed by A.C. Masquelet *"A thought that one cannot express correctly will be difficult to implement"* and by E. Morscher:

"The absence of planning is the planning of a failure".

Third Part: Surgical Technique

The implantation of a prosthesis must never be considered as a succession of "tips and tricks" or other "recipes" which, taken together, will lead to a successful surgery. Such reasoning, or rather not reasoning, would certainly entail a long learning period or even a chronic incapacity to perform a surgical act correctly. An operating technique must be adapted to the chosen concept, and the purpose of every surgical gesture must be clearly formulated and understood by the surgeon.

Fourth Part: Evaluation of the Radiographic Results – How?

The methods for clinical evaluation are known and admitted by all authors. By contrast, the radiographic evaluation is a domain where confusion reigns. To our knowledge, no method achieves the double objective of evaluating the bone stock surrounding an implant while at the same time assessing the quality of osseointegration and secondary stability. At the time of the study of the results of an implant, the evaluation of the radiographic results constitutes a "weak link".

Fifth Part: Evaluation of the Radiographic Results – Why?

Evaluating the radiographic results enables the surgeon to identify the direction to follow to improve his own results and those of his colleagues because a surgeon must share his own experience and every operator must benefit from the experience of all!

Part I

Press-Fit Concept

In joint replacement surgery, little space is devoted to the understanding and good use of an implant, or it is reduced to a few, unspecific sentences. The consequence of this inevitably results in difficulties during surgery and in clinical results that do not always meet the surgeon's expectations. Furthermore, it makes the transmission of experience uncertain.

Choice of a Concept

Every surgeon makes a choice based on his own convictions. Being an advocate of an uncemented concept does not exclude the possibility of using cement in specific situations. Furthermore, justifying the choice of an uncemented prosthesis by condemning cement (or vice versa) is inefficient and often only leads to the revival of a debate which regularly opposes advocates of either method.

In the case of revision, however, there seems to be less controversy as it is known that an uncemented implant in revision surgery often does not require additional grafts if primary stability in good conditions can be achieved. Such an undertaking is not always possible with a cemented prosthesis.

All uncemented concepts, however, are not equal, and it is advisable to be well informed before making a choice.

The Press-Fit Concept

While effective, the press-fit concept is also demanding and it must be rigorously applied in every situation. Besides, achieving primary stability is not the only objective when an uncemented implant is chosen. It is also necessary to protect the surrounding bone and to promote its regeneration in the longer term, if it is affected. In the case of an uncemented femoral stem, this means choosing a well designed prosthesis and using efficient instruments to achieve proximal fixation, whenever possible, or to implant a short stem when primary stability is sought in the diaphyseal region. The latter is often the case in revision situations.

The Uncemented Concepts: Parameters to Make a Reasoned Choice

When choosing an uncemented femoral stem, it is wise to decide exclusively on the basis of the concept. This is the only way to select, among the numerous prostheses proposed to a surgeon, the implant which offers the best compromise.

A concept without cement must be well defined, with clear objectives that are easy to achieve during surgery. A poorly defined concept is always difficult to implement in surgical practice.

1.1 What Must Be Avoided

Concepts That Are "Too Innovative"

The concept of such implants is not clearly established; the main objective is to follow a fashion trend. The advent of minimally invasive surgery constitutes a good example of what can happen under such circumstances: the top priority is no longer the primary stability of the implant but the challenge of designing a prosthesis that can be introduced in the medullary cavity through a minimal skin incision via the femoral neck. And, thus, we can observe the birth of prostheses with an unexpected design – to say the least – and whose primary stability is impossible to achieve in every case.

For the moment, implants intended for revisions escape this trend. We can only hope that designing surgeons and manufacturers will continue to act wisely and carefully!

1.2 What Is Preferable to Avoid

The "Copies"

A copy is an implant (often for first intention) which is the result of a modification, sometimes discreet, of the geometrical characteristics of a prosthesis which has already proven its efficiency and which is a simple imitation. These pseudo-innovations can be dangerous because a modification, even small, can have consequences with regard to biomechanics. This really turns the copy into a "new" prosthesis, likely to give less good results than the original model.

The optimal geometry as well as the nature of the materials for a purposeful concept are well known. To deviate from designs which have proven their efficiency over several years, under the pretext of being innovative, represents an unnecessary risk.

1.3 What Needs to Be Considered with Caution

1.3.1 Modular Implants

At the time of choosing an implant of this type, the surgeon must have two considerations in mind: (1) Regardless of the performance of the manufacturer, an assembly system represents a zone of increased fragility and, in this regard, the objective is not to eliminate all possible risks but to reduce them to a minimum. (2) Certain assembly systems, designed by unscrupulous manufacturers, are programmed to break after a short time. A marketing authorization does not constitute a sufficient safeguard !

When choosing a modular implant, it is recommended to verify with the manufacturer the guarantees of reliability offered by the proposed assembly system. Besides, be aware that modularity is not in itself a concept for ensuring the primary stability of an implant, but rather a characteristic of manufacturing which allows a rigorous application of the press-fit concept (see Chap. 4)

1.3.2 The "Mixed" Concepts

This is a combination of several different concepts for the same implant in the hope of ensuring reliable primary stability. The most typical example is a femoral revision stem

P. Le Béguec et al., *Uncemented Femoral Stems for Revision Surgery*,
DOI 10.1007/978-3-319-03614-4_1, © Springer International Publishing Switzerland 2015

which would be at the same time anatomical (i.e. curved), intended for self-locking, and whose stability could also be achieved by press-fit. This invites several remarks:

- Firstly, the curvature of a femoral stem can only be used in one plane, usually the sagittal plane, and if the femur is also curved in the frontal plane (which is often the case in revision), this geometrical characteristic is of no interest.
- Secondly, proximal fixation is not possible with this type of implant, which is a real handicap, especially in the case of an osteoporotic femur.
- Thirdly, if a diaphyseal fixation is indicated, it is always difficult to adapt the curvature of the femur to that of the implant. Primary stability is often achieved by means of a 3-point support, which can prove insufficient to neutralize the rotational forces what makes the locking quasi-mandatory. Fourthly, making a stem "self-locking" always has a weakening effect on the implant, which means that this characteristic can only be applied to implants of sufficient diameter and with a rather cylindrical configuration, and thus more invasive.

In the end, the drawbacks of each of these concepts have a tendency to add up more than the advantages; overall, these implants do not offer increased security.

1.4 What Is Possible But in Limited Indications

1.4.1 Use of a Primary Stem for Revision Surgery

If an implant has proven its efficiency in primary surgery, it can also be valid for revisions. Yet, the number of cases which can benefit from such implants is limited, even if the stem was lengthened, and the surgeon should always have a prosthesis more particularly intended for revision available.

1.4.2 Stems with Distal Locking

These prostheses have proven their efficiency when fixation at the level of the distal third of the femur is the only possibility. In daily practice, these cases are rare, and in so-called normal or intermediate situations, we voice some criticism against this concept: primary stability can only be diaphyseal (isthmus or distal femur), and proximal fixation is not possible; a long stem is inevitable even when it is not indispensable; there is a risk of fracture for stems with a diameter of less than 18 mm; the transmission of bending constraints is highly perturbed, and, theoretically, makes unlocking always

necessary; finally, when the cortices are weakened by osteoporosis, the quality of the locking is questionable.

1.4.3 Custom-Made Stems

In reality, there are only few inevitable indications in primary or revision surgery. Especially, the manufacturing limitations are too significant and costly to advocate the use of this concept in daily practice.

It also has to be pointed out that if the design corresponds exactly with the endomedullary cavity – which should theoretically always be the case – these implants are also, by definition, invasive and increase the risk of stress-shielding.

1.5 Frequently Used Uncemented Concepts

The following two concepts are often used and show similarities:

1.5.1 The "Fit and Fill" Concept

This concept is often marked by femoral stems with extensive porous coating, a straight configuration and a globally cylindrical cross-section. These implants are intended to bridge the proximal loss of bone stock. Primary stability is ensured by an intimate contact between the "recipient" femur and the implant, over a distance of several centimeters and at the level of the isthmic zone of the femur.

1.5.2 The "Press-Fit" Concept

This concept features stems of straight and tapered configuration. Primary stability is ensured by means of a bone-implant surface contact and generation of a pretension (or prestressing) that is higher than the destabilizing forces (subsidence and rotation) at the level of the bone/implant interface.

These two concepts take into account biomechanical features clearly established, and can ensure primary stability efficiently; on the other hand, their inconvenience is an increased risk of stress shielding, in particular if the bone/implant contact area is extensive, which, by definition, is always the case with the "fit and fill" concept. This inconvenience can often be minimized with the press-fit concept, and it is primarily for that reason that we have opted for this concept.

Conclusion

The most important objective for an uncemented femoral prosthesis is to ensure primary stability. To achieve this first goal, all concepts do not offer the same efficiency. This is especially true for femoral stems dedicated to revision.

Furthermore, it is necessary to avoid implantation of a prosthesis that is too invasive. This has several drawbacks: degradation of the bone stock due to stress-shielding if the stem has a circular cross-section and if it is long: imperfect proximal osseointegration or difficult ablation with risk of serious damage to the bone stock if the stem is not loose. To minimize such risks, it is necessary to choose a concept and an implant system which:

- Does not fill the entire endomedullary space and thus does not stiffen the surrounding bone too much;
- Can achieve proximal primary stability whenever possible;

Offers a short stem for situations where primary stability needs to be in the diaphyseal region. A short stem will also always be easier to extract, should this become necessary.

"To describe a concept is also to define the main characteristics of an implant"

In the prosthetic industry, press-fit is a concept that is frequently used to mechanically assemble two separate elements. In surgical practice, Zweymüller et al. [1] was one of the first to use press-fit to ensure the primary stability of an uncemented femoral in primary surgery. In 1987, Wagner [2] introduced this concept to revision stems, and since then, several surgeons have followed the same path [3, 4]. However, and in spite of very widespread usage, it appears that most surgeons are not familiar with the principles of the press-fit concept. This lack of knowledge explains, for the most part, its poor application in surgical practice. To find a solution for this knowledge gap, it is necessary to recall the principles of this concept. This gives us a better understanding of the conditions that need to be fulfilled to obtain a real press-fit effect in surgical practice.

2.1 Principles of the Press-Fit Concept

To obtain a press-fit effect (be it in primary or revision surgery), it is necessary to generate a pretension (or prestressing) at the level of the bone/implant interface. In the case of a femoral stem, this means provoking a pressure superior to destabilizing forces such as the constraints in subsidence and rotation.

Morscher [5, 6] states that two requirements are necessary to ensure a surgical press-fit effect: (1) obtain a cortical bone/implant surface contact (Fig. 2.1a) and (2) ensure perfect wedging of the implant (Fig. 2.1b).

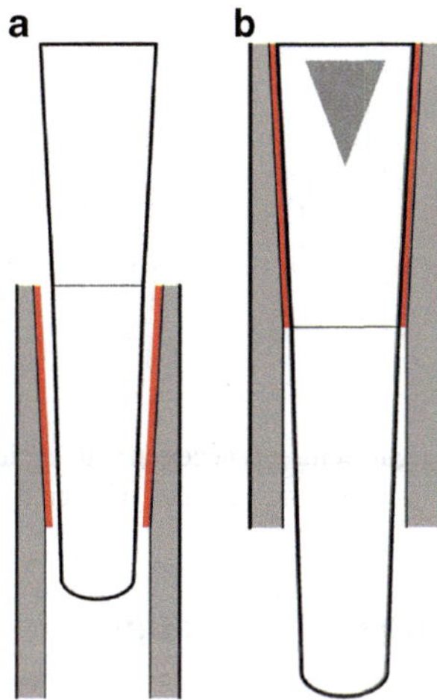

Fig. 2.1 The press-fit concept requires: (**a**) remodeling of the endomedullary spacc to obtain a cortical bone/implant surface contact; (**b**) wedging of an implant with the same geometrical configuration in this space

If these two conditions, that are indispensable for a true press-fit effect, are ignored by the surgeon, there is little chance that these two parameters will be correctly applied during surgery.

2.1.1 Bone/Implant Contact

A *straight stem* is the safest means to ensure a cortical bone/implant contact in the form of a surface. But, with such an implant, it is necessary to avoid a 3-point support, what, in practice, means:

P. Le Béguec et al., *Uncemented Femoral Stems for Revision Surgery*,
DOI 10.1007/978-3-319-03614-4_2, © Springer International Publishing Switzerland 2015

- Avoid varus implantation. This risk is always present when an endofemoral approach is chosen, even if the femur is straight in the frontal plane (Fig. 2.2a).
- Take into account the presence of a femoral curvature and perform a femoral osteotomy (in the form of a trochanteric-diaphyseal flap) when the femur is curved, which is not uncommon during a revision (Fig. 2.2b).

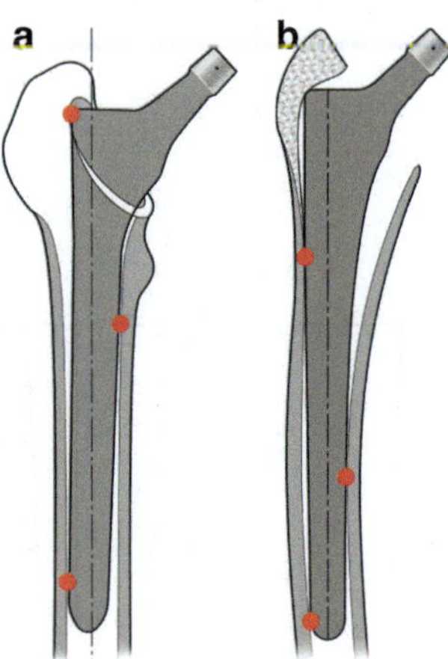

Fig. 2.2 With a straight stem, it is necessary: to avoid a varus implantation (**a**); to take into account the presence of a femoral curvature (**b**)

2.1.2 Wedging of the Implant

Wedging an implant means ensuring primary stability by creating a pretension at the level of the bone/implant interface. To obtain good wedging, an implant with a *tapered configuration* offers two advantages:
- Generation of a stabilizing horizontal force
- Progressive decrease (from top to bottom) of the vertical shearing stress

These two biomechanical characteristics of a tapered shape, as described by Kerboull [7] for cemented stems, also applies to uncemented stems (Fig. 2.3).

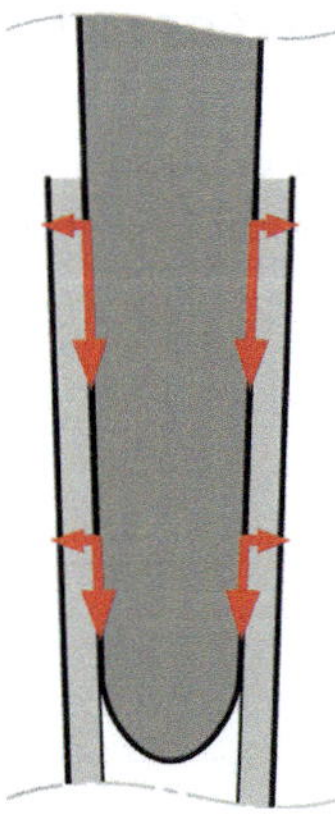

Fig. 2.3 A tapered configuration to develop a horizontal compressive force

2.2 "Press-Fit*able*" Zones

The press-fit concept can be applied:
1. At the level of the proximal femur where it is possible to define a metaphyseal (zone a) and a metaphyseal-diaphyseal (zone b).
2. In the diaphyseal region (femoral isthmus) (Fig. 2.4).

   A press-fit cannot be achieved in the distal third of the femur if the medullary cavity widens

   A press-fit is defined as:
- Proximal, when it is achieved in zones 1a and/or b.
- Diaphyseal, if it occurs in zone 2.
- Global, when it occurs in both, zones 1 and 2.

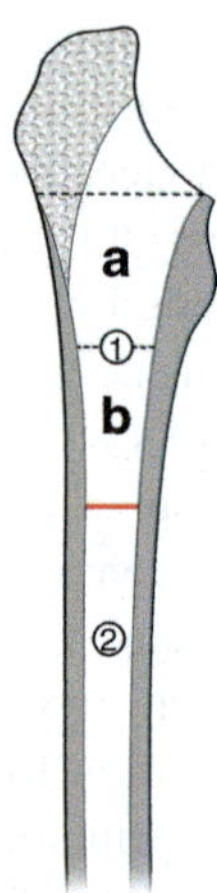

Fig. 2.4 The various "press-fit*able*" zones

2.2.1 Proximal Press-Fit

2.2.1.1 Metaphyseal Zone (Zone 1a)
This zone is situated between the tip of the greater trochanter and the base of the lesser trochanter. In revision surgery, a press-fit effect in the metaphyseal zone is possible only if the bone stock is preserved.
- In the frontal plane (Fig. 2.5), it is difficult to regularly obtain support on the medial cortex (Merkel) and there is often no spongy tissue in this zone of the femur.

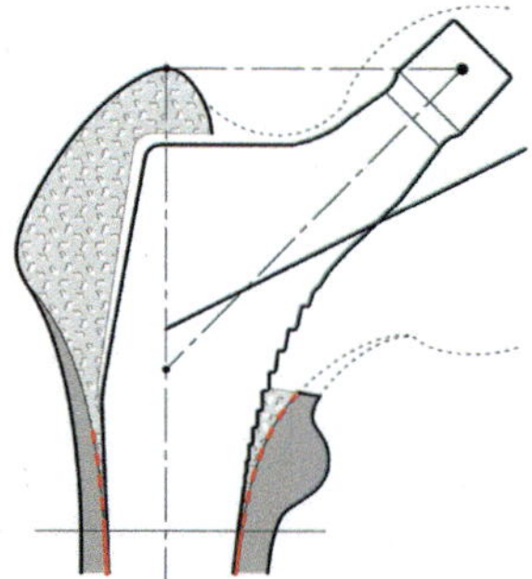

Fig. 2.5 In revision surgery, it is difficult to achieve a true press-fit effect in the frontal plane of the metayseal region

- In the sagittal plane (Fig. 2.6), a press-fit effect can be envisaged only with an ad hoc implant.

A bone/implant contact over the entire distance of the posterior cortex is often possible. At the level of the anterior cortex, contact is only possible over a short distance because of the frequent presence of an antecurvatum in the proximal femur.

Thus, to ensure a press-fit in the sagittal plane, it is often necessary to preserve the cancellous bone tissue or to insert endomedullary grafts at the level of the anterior metaphyseal zone.

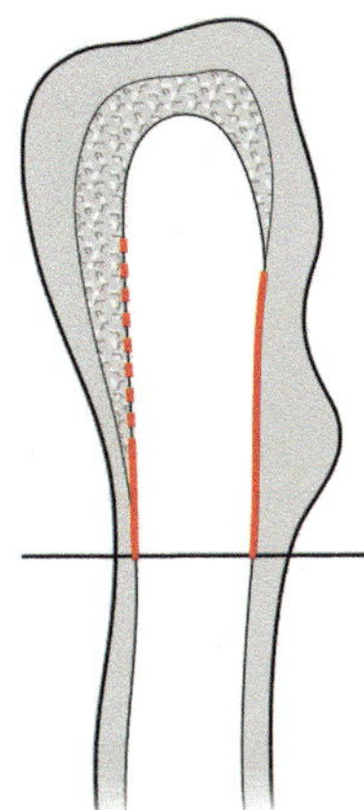

Fig. 2.6   Metaphyseal support in the sagittal plane

2.2.1.2 Metaphyseo-Diaphyseal Zone (Zone 1b)

This is a naturally tapered space which is situated immediately below the lesser trochanter. In many cases, endocortical support can be obtained at this level over a distance of 2–3 cm, in both the frontal (Fig. 2.7a) and sagittal (Fig. 2.7b) planes.

In revision surgery, if that the bone stock is preserved and the femur straight, this zone of the proximal femur can safely be used for the primary stability of an uncemented implant.

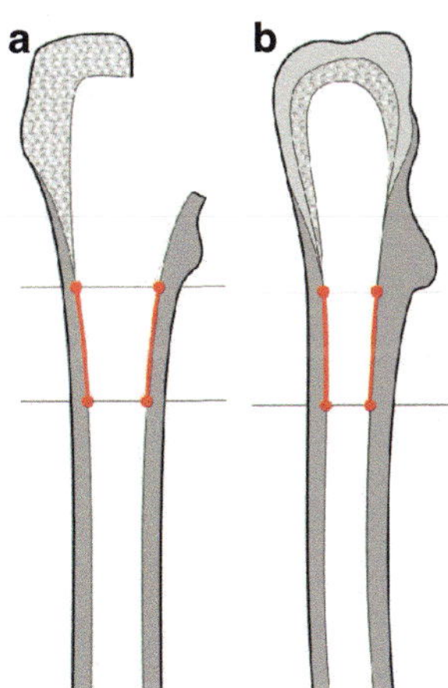

Fig. 2.7   A metaphyseo-diaphyseal press-fit can be obtained. In the frontal plane (**a**). In the sagittal plane (**b**)

2.2.2   Diaphyseal Press-Fit

A diaphyseal press-fit is mandatory when a femoral flap is performed, which is often the case in revision surgery (Fig. 2.8). In such a situation, the objective is always to achieve a bone/implant surface contact over a short distance of approximately 3 cm at the level of the isthmic zone. Contrary to Wagner [2], we think that a bone/implant contact over a longer distance (5 cm) is difficult to achieve, most often unnecessary and possibly even harmful (risk of stress-shielding).

Reminder. If the femoral isthmus is destroyed, the press-fit concept cannot be used.

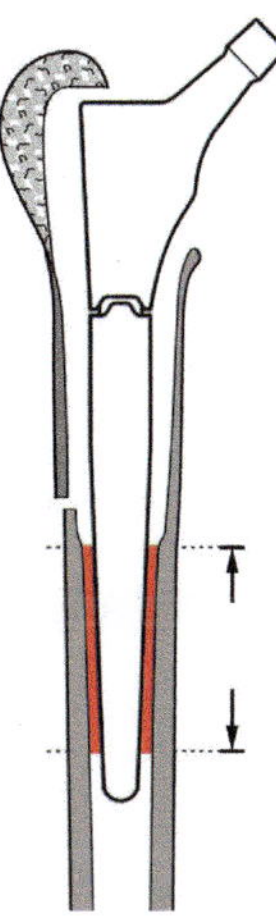

Fig. 2.8   Diaphyseal press-fit in the isthmic zone after performing a femoral flap

The Press-Fit Concept: Practical Application

In practice, within the framework of a revision, the press-fit can be proximal in the metaphyseo-diaphyseal zone or diaphyseal in the isthmic zone.

There are two particular cases: a global press-fit (i.e. at the same time proximal and diaphyseal) and a proximal press-fit on a femoral flap.

Independent of the chosen zone, bi-cortical support – at least in the frontal or sagittal plane – and over a short distance of approximately 3 cm should be sought to ensure reliable press-fit.

3.1 How to Ensure a Proximal Press-Fit?

A proximal press-fit, most often in the metaphyseo-diaphyseal region, must be aimed for (or discussed) whenever the femur is straight in the frontal plane and when there are no or only small bone defects in Gruen zone(s) 2 and/or 6.

3.1.1 Femoral Approach

An endofemoral approach is the rule, with a *wide lateral and posterior opening* of the greater trochanter, to ensure that you are working in the femoral axis (Fig. 3.1a, b).

Insufficient opening of the greater trochanter always entails a varus implantation, which makes a bone/implant surface contact and, consequently, a true press-fit effect impossible.

When choosing a straight press-fit stem, the opening of the greater trochanter is an important step in the surgical procedure that must never be neglected. It is recommended to be particularly vigilant at this point of the intervention, as this

zone of the femur is often very dense, sclerotic or difficult to remodel in revision situations.

Nb. A trochanteric osteotomy keeps its indications when a straight stem is chosen. It allows primarily to eliminate proximal obstacles (proximal curvature of the femur after osteotomy) and it can facilitate proximal fixation of the implant.

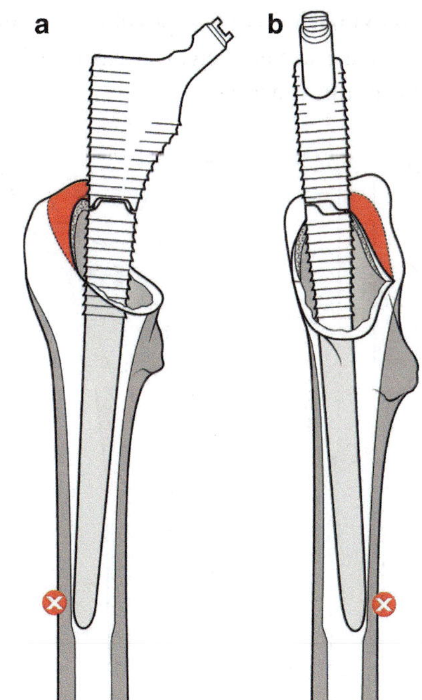

Fig. 3.1 Remodeling of the greater trochanter. Lateral opening (**a**). Posterior opening (often neglected) (**b**)

P. Le Béguec et al., *Uncemented Femoral Stems for Revision Surgery*,
DOI 10.1007/978-3-319-03614-4_3, © Springer International Publishing Switzerland 2015

3.1.2 Preparation of a Proximal Anchorage Zone

- Metaphyseal anchorage (zone 1a). The preparation is usually performed with a rasp that also serves as trial prosthesis. Gradually increase the size of the rasp, which is in a monobloc form if it is a modular rasp. Preserve the cancellous bone at the level of the anterior metaphyseal zone or, as often necessary, insert bone grafts at this level of the femur.
  This anchorage mode is rarely possible in revision.
- Metaphyseo-diaphyseal anchorage (zone 1b). In revision surgery, it is always difficult to accurately plan the zone of primary stability in this region of the femur prior to surgery. Preparation in two steps with a modular rasp ensures that you are always at the right level (Fig. 3.2a, b).

NB. The preparation of a proximal anchorage zone can also be achieved with a long reamer that is moreover useful to adjust or complete the lateral and posterior opening of the greater trochanter. A trial rasp-prosthesis remains, however, indispensable to finalize the preparation of the inter-trochanteric zone and to choose the final implant.

When a proximal press-fit is possible, wedging of the final implant at the correct height is easily achieved after inserting bone grafts, if necessary.

3.2 How to Ensure a Diaphyseal Press-Fit?

3.2.1 Femoral Approach

*A **trochantero-diaphyseal flap*** is the rule when the press-fit zone needs to be situated in the diaphyseal region (isthmic zone) (Fig. 3.3a).

The primary objective is to be near to a well corticalized and straight segment of the femur, knowing that *reamers cannot make a curved femur straight, especially when reaming from a distance !*

A lateral trochantero-diaphyseal flap is often combined with an osteotomy of the medial cortex *(bi-cortical osteotomy)* to reduce a femoral curvature in the sagittal plane which is often an obstacle to the preparation of the anchorage zone in the form of a surface (Fig. 3.3b). If the quality of the cortices is good and the cortices are in close contact with the implant at the end of the surgery, this osteotomy makes it furthermore possible to enhance primary stability of the implant and favoring proximal secondary osseointegration.

NB. By an endofemoral approach we can only complete or secure, in diaphyseal region, a proximal precarious anchoring (bone defects localized in zones 2 and/or 6)

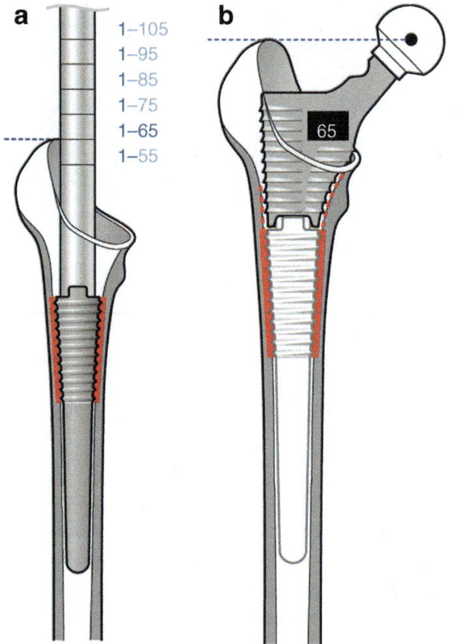

Fig. 3.2 A modular rasp to a preparation in two steps: Preparation of the metaphyseo-diaphyseal anchorage zone (**a**). Metaphyseal preparation and choice of the implant (**b**)

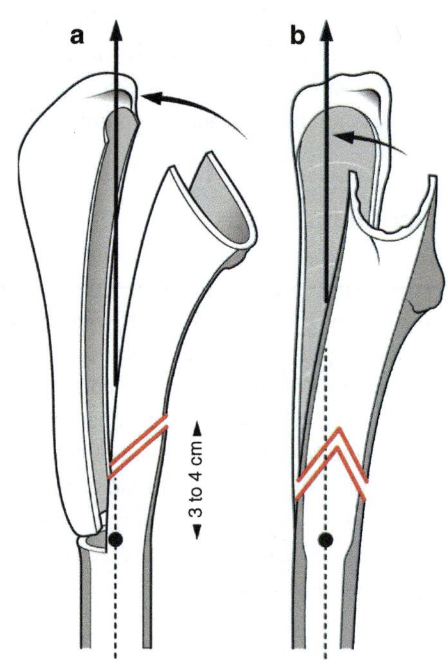

Fig. 3.3 If the femur is curved, a bi-cortical osteotomy is necessary in the front plans (**a**) and the sagittal plane (**b**)

3.2.2   Preparation of a Diaphyseal Anchorage Zone

The preparation of the isthmic anchorage zone is performed with a reamer whose sole function is the reshaping of the medullary cavity to give it the same configuration as that of the selected implant, i.e. tapered, in most cases (Fig. 3.4a).

To be efficient, it is necessary to be *near the anchorage zone and ream a straight segment of the femur over a short distance*. It is difficult to make a medullary cavity tapered over a distance of more than 3 cm, especially when the cortices are thick (Fig. 3.4b).

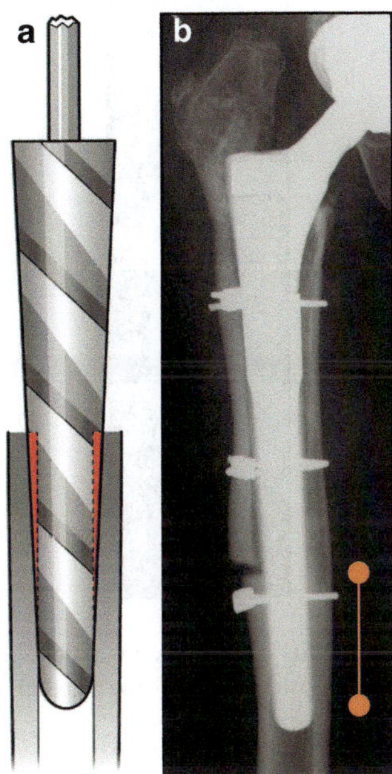

Fig. 3.4   Reamers to give the femur a conical configuration over a short distance (**a**) and to ensure a short effect press-fit (**b**)

3.2.3   Selection of the Implant with a Trial Prosthesis

The objective is to keep a "conical reserve", which is a guarantee for a perfect wedging while making re-wedging possible (Fig. 3.5).

In every case, it is thus necessary to ensure primary stability in the distal or intermediate part of the tapered zone of the implant.

It is impossible to choose the "right" implant with a reamer

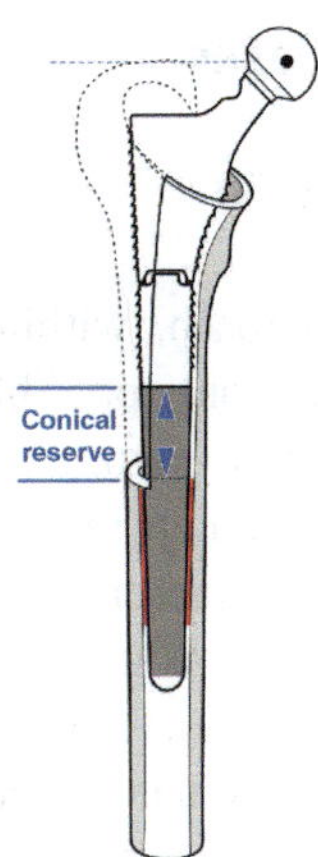

Fig. 3.5   A trial prosthesis is indispensable for the selection of an implant with a "conical reserve"

3.2.4   Insertion and Wedging of the Final Stem in Two Steps

- If the femur has been prepared carefully with the ad hoc instruments, wedging of the definitive implant usually occurs at the same level as that of the trial prosthesis. In these circumstances, implantation of the final stem can be done in one step once the two prosthetic components have been assembled outside of the femur.
- Implantation in two steps is possible with a modular prosthesis. (1) Implantation of the distal component of the final implant with a provisional proximal component (Fig. 3.6a) (2) Selection and assembling of the final proximal component whose length restores the correct length of the lower limb (Fig. 3.6b).

We strongly warn against implantation in two steps without performing a femoral flap

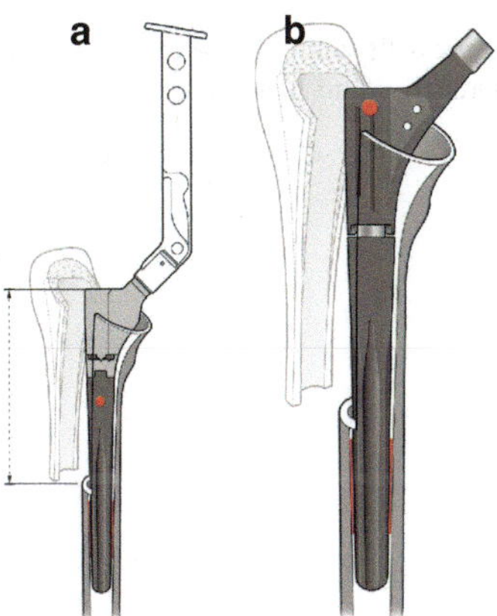

Fig. 3.6   An implantation in two steps: Implantation of the distal part (**a**). Selection and assembly of the definitive proximal part (**b**)

3.3   Particular Cases

3.3.1   Global Press-Fit

- By endofemoral approach, within the framework of a revision, this option is only possible if there are no bone defects and if the femur is straight. This is the guarantee for perfect primary stability (Fig. 3.7a)
  NB. With regard to the preservation of bone stock in the long term, this method of fixation does not present a risk in the absence of osteoporosis. On the other hand, in the presence of osteoporosis – even in its early stages – it is always preferable to avoid diaphyseal fixation whenever possible.
- When a femoral flap has been performed, a diaphyseal press-fit can be extended to the proximal femur if the cortices are of a good quality and close to the implant (Fig. 3.7b).

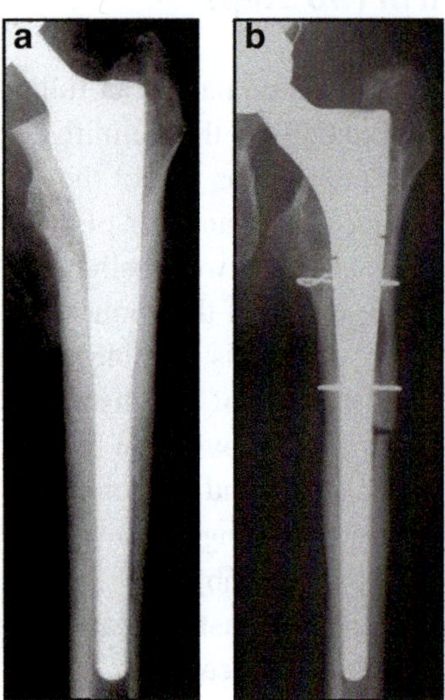

Fig. 3.7 Global press-fit within the framework of a revision. (**a**) By endofemoral approach, if no bone defects. (**b**) After femoral flap, if good cortices

3.3.2   Proximal Press-Fit by Means of a Flap

This option can ensure the primary stability of an uncemented stem while favoring proximal transmission of bending stresses. One condition is necessary: the cortices (medial and lateral) must be in close contact with the implant and of sufficient quality to allow efficient cerclage wiring (Fig. 3.8).

- **This is also an interesting approach "to globalize" a somewhat precarious diaphyseal press-fit and, thus, to avoid the implantation of a longer stem**

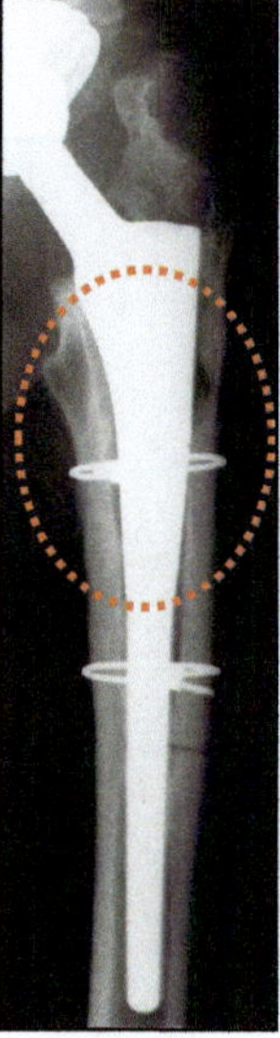

Fig. 3.8 Proximal stability by means of a flap: remodeling of the greater trochanter and osteotomy of the medial cortex are often necessary

The objective of this chapter is not to give an exhaustive review of the various geometrical shapes that can produce a press-fit effect, but to give the surgeon some clues on how to choose the implant that offers the best compromise.

> **Warnings**
>
> The comments developed below are not preconceived notions against a particular type of implant. It is important to avoid polemics whose only goal is to silence those who think differently. Thus, in revision surgery, so-called "curved" stems have also demonstrated their efficiency. Moreover, they can be indicated in certain situations. We estimate, however, that within the framework of the press-fit concept, it is possible to proceed otherwise and, above all, to do better with a straight stem.

4.1 General Considerations

4.1.1 The Nature of Materials and Implant Surfaces

Today, we have good knowledge of these two areas; it is just important to remember that an osseoinductive (or osseoconductive) coating does not, in itself, constitute a concept to assure primary stability for an uncemented implant; it is one characteristic, among others, that can facilitate secondary osseointegration.

4.1.2 Primary Stability and Loads Transmission

A surgeon who opts for an uncemented concept has to conciliate two conflicting objectives: ensuring the primary stability of the chosen implant without compromising the transmission of bending stresses (tensile and compressive forces) to minimize the risk of stress shielding.

To reach such an objective, there is only one possibility: not fill the endomedullary space too much. In order to do this, one should locate the endomedullary supports, i.e. the press-fit zone, at the level of the neutral zone of the femur. According to the work of Blaimont et al. [8], this zone is situated at the intersection of the tensile and compressive forces, i.e. in the sagittal plane at the level of the proximal femur and in the frontal plane at the level of the diaphyseal femur (Fig. 4.1)

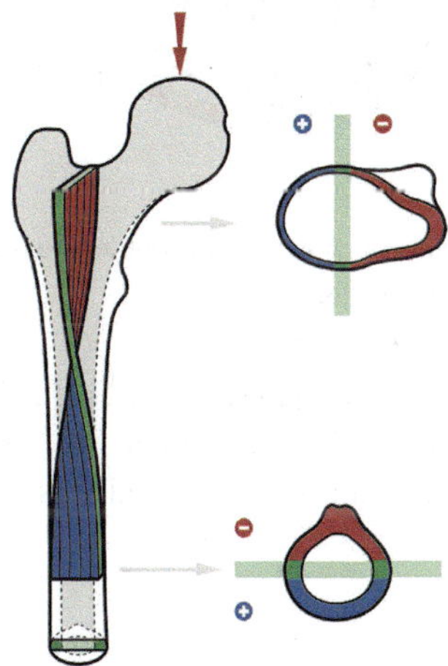

Fig. 4.1 Bending stresses and the neutral zone of the femur

4.1.3 Modularity

As suggested by Essig and Puget as early as 1995 [9], modularity, which is often used for revision prostheses, offers a large range of stems but also has a drawback: independent of the manufacturing technique used, modularity always weakens an implant. It is also necessary to remember that modularity is not a concept to ensure primary stability of an uncemented implant in itself. On the other hand, modular ancillary instruments offer decisive advantages in the case of the press-fit concept because they facilitate the preparation of the anchoring zone and the selection of the correct implant.

P. Le Béguec et al., *Uncemented Femoral Stems for Revision Surgery*,
DOI 10.1007/978-3-319-03614-4_4, © Springer International Publishing Switzerland 2015

4.2 Main Characteristics of a Press-Fit Implant and Instruments

4.2.1 Proximal Press-Fit

To ensure a proximal press-fit, a straight and tapered stem (frontal and sagittal plane) constitutes a good compromise. In the horizontal plane, a globally quadrangular cross-section is also efficient, with possible variations depending on the zone concerned (metaphyseal or metaphyseo-diaphyseal).

4.2.1.1 Implant for Proximal Press-Fit

- In the metaphyseal zone, when the cortices are present, a wide implant in the sagittal plane is necessary to ensure a support on the cortices (Fig. 4.2).

  Reminder. At the level of the anterior metaphyseal zone, it is necessary to preserve the cancellous bone or to add cortico-spongious grafts if a support on the cortex is not possible, which is often the case.

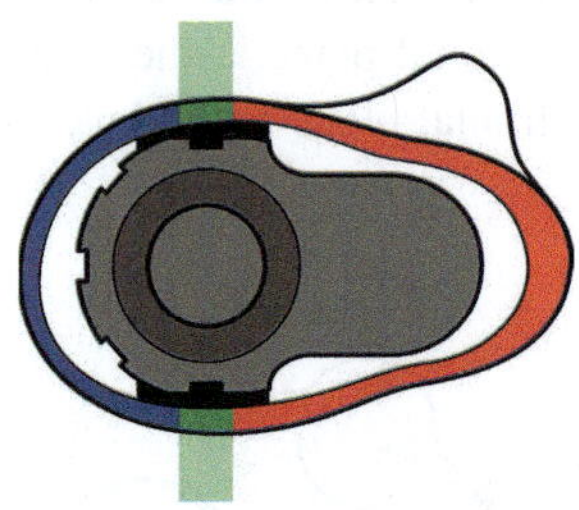

Fig. 4.2 An implant which is wide in profile to ensure a metaphyseal press-fit in the sagittal plane

- In the metaphyseo-diaphyseal zone, a quadrangular cross-section, or one with longitudinal fins, avoids excessive filling of the medullary canal and allows a good control of the rotational forces (Fig. 4.3).

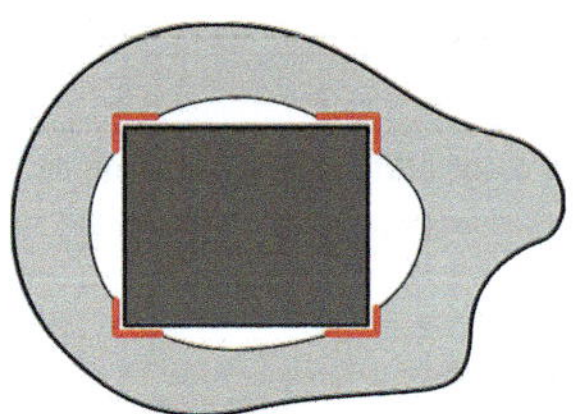

Fig. 4.3 A quadrangular configuration in the metaphyseo-diaphyseal zone

4.2.1.2 Ancillary Instruments for Proximal Press-Fit

A modular rasp® (Fig. 4.4a), which also serves as trial prosthesis, helps to prepare the press-fit anchorage zone at the right level. This instrument also compensates for the drawback of a monobloc rasp which can remain stuck in the upper metaphyseal zone (Fig. 4.4b).

A modular rasp® facilitates achieving proximal press-fit while avoiding a diaphyseal fixation that is too tight, thus decreasing the risk of stress-shielding in the presence of osteoporosis.

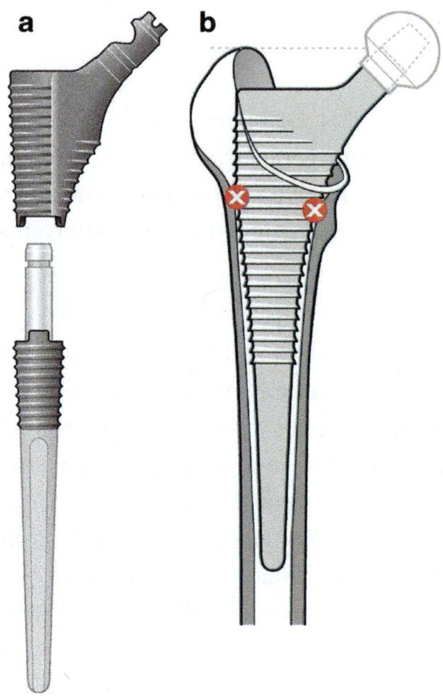

Fig. 4.4 Instruments for proximal press-fit: modular rasp to prepare the anchorage zone at the right level (**a**), what is not always possible with a monobloc rasp (**b**)

4.2.2 Diaphyseal Press-Fit

- First objective: obtain a bone/implant surface contact with a short stem and avoid excessive filling of the medullary cavity.
- Second objective: ensure perfect wedging.

4.2.2.1 Implant for Diaphyseal Press-Fit

- **A straight stem**: to ensure a surface contact, because *it is always easier to straighten a femur rather than adapt its curvature to that of an implant.*

To ensure a bone/implant surface contact in the diaphyseal region, the choice of a curved stem can seem coherent upon first analysis, as the femur is mostly curved in the sagittal plane. This assertion, which seems at first glance irrefutable, is in reality debatable, and this for two reasons:

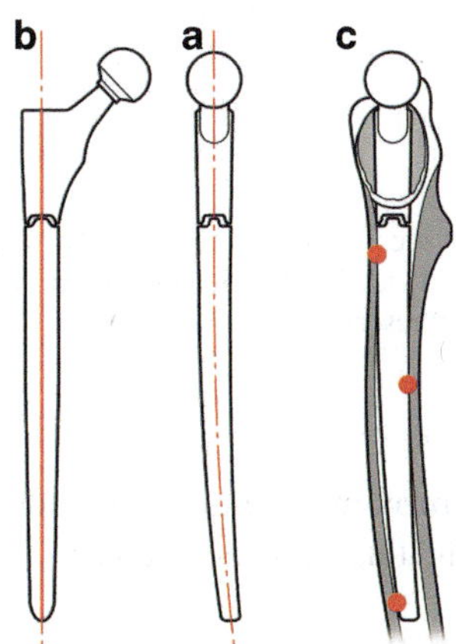

Fig. 4.5 Characteristics of a curved stem: The curvature of this type of stem is in the sagittal plane (**a**). A curved stem in profile is straight in the frontal view (**b**). A curved stem usually stabilizes by means of a three-point support (**c**)

- The curvature of these implants can only be used in the sagittal plane (Fig. 4.5a). Therefore, a curved stem in profile is straight in the frontal view (Fig. 4.5b). This does not allow it to escape the constraints imposed by a femoral curvature in the frontal plane, i.e. the necessity to perform a femoral osteotomy.
- The curvature of these implants rarely matches the curvature of the femur (Fig. 4.5c) and it is impossible to ensure a surface contact between bone and implant with a rasp.
- **A not very invasive stem**: *avoid a stem of circular section in the diaphyseal region*, which could entail a deviation of the loads, and opt for an implant that ensures bone/implant contact only in the frontal plane (Fig. 4.6).

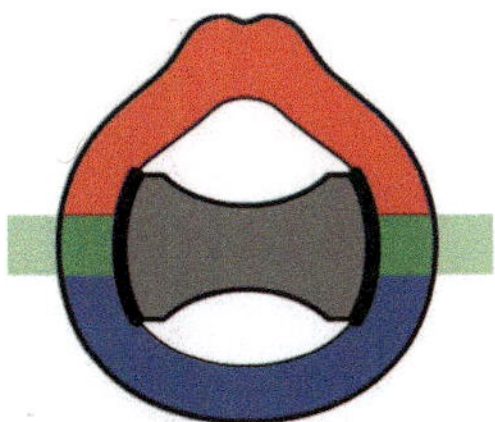

Fig. 4.6 Characteristics of a stem which is not too invasive in the diaphyseal region: Ensure a bone/implant contact in the frontal plane.

A stem with longitudinal fins (Fig. 4.7a) or with a quadrangular configuration (Fig. 4.7b) allows you to achieve this objective. Moreover, these two implant configurations ensure good control of the rotational constraints, which are not always easy to neutralize with an uncemented implant.

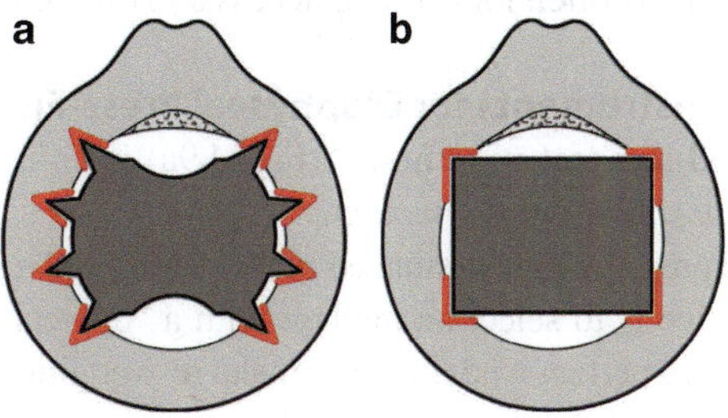

Fig. 4.7 Stem with longitudinal fins (**a**) or Quadrangular stem (**b**)

- **A tapered stem**: to facilitate wedging of the implant and making re-wedging possible. This eliminates the risk of a significant secondary subsidence if the anchorage zone was not carefully prepared or if the wedging was insufficient.

The reamers, which are intended to make the medullary cavity conical, should be particularly effective because it is never easy to make a medullary cavity conical when the cortices are dense and thick

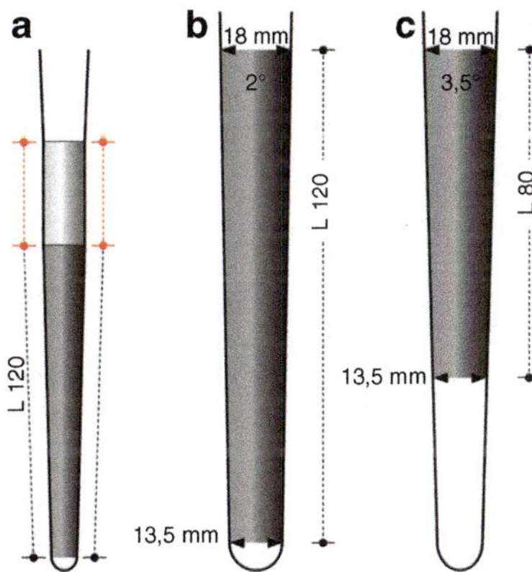

Fig. 4.8 Geometric characteristics of a tapered stem: A long tapered stem always has a cylindrical segment (**a**). Small taper angle of 2°: entire tapered zone is usable (**b**). Bigger taper angle of 3. 5°: the distal tapered zone is unusable (**c**)

A tapered configuration entails geometrical characteristics. The surgeon must be aware of them when making a choice and when wedging the final implant into place.

- A tapered revision stem, when it is long, always includes a cylindrical segment which is not favorable to wedging or re-wedging (Fig. 4.8a).
- A small taper angle can make wedging of the implant more delicate; but this geometrical configuration has the advantage of increasing the height of the tapered zone, and the distal part of these implants can be used without any risk for the implantation of a short stem (Fig. 4.8b).

- Inversely, the more accentuated the taper angle, the easier and safer the wedging. But, this geometric shape also has two inconveniences: the height of the tapered zone is shorter and the diameter of the distal part of the implant is reduced, which makes this zone unusable and imposes a stem that is often longer than necessary (Fig. 4.8c).

4.2.2.2 Instruments for Diaphyseal Press-Fit

- **A modular test prosthesis**® (Fig. 4.9a) is *indispensable to choosing the right implant*.

  If the press-fit zone is situated in the diaphyseal region, the objective is to select an implant with a "conical reserve" to ensure perfect wedging or to make re-wedging possible.

  If the stability is ensured by the tapered proximal zone, it is often possible to increase the diameter of the implant without modifying the diameter of the medullary canal. This is achieved by choosing a shorter stem to avoid a length discrepancy between the two lower limbs (Fig. 4.9b). Thus, modular instruments are also an excellent means to opt for a short stem!

  Choosing the "right" implant is impossible with a reamer

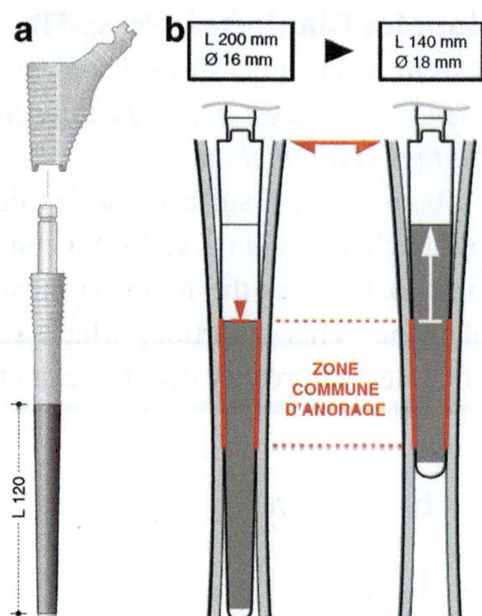

Fig. 4.9 Characteristics of a test prosthesis: The tapered portion must be clearly delineated (**a**). Modularity facilitates the choice of a short stem with a "conical reserve" (**b**)

- **Temporary proximal component**® for implantation in two steps if the final stem is modular.

The most important objective for an uncemented femoral prosthesis is to ensure primary stability. To achieve this first goal, all concepts do not offer the same efficiency. This is especially true for femoral stems dedicated to revision.

The Press-Fit Concept

- The press-fit concept is a reliable means to ensure the primary stability of an uncemented femoral stem provided we respect two very precise rules (1) Obtain a bone/implant surface contact (2) Ensure a perfect wedging of the implant.
- To be effective during the preparation of the femur, it is necessary to be near the anchorage zone which, in many cases, necessitates a femoral flap when the press-fit zone is in the diaphyseal region.

The Implant

Generally speaking, an implant can be considered as safe when it presents the characteristics which make it possible to reach the goals imposed by the chosen concept. In the case of the press-fit concept, a straight stem and of tapered configuration constitutes a good compromise to ensure primary stability. It is also necessary to choose a stem that can achieve proximal primary stability whenever possible and, when the primary stability needs to be in the diaphyseal region, to choose an implant which is not too long and does not stiffen the surrounding bone too much (stem with circular cross-section). Such implant has two drawbacks: degradation of the bone stock due to stress shielding and imperfect proximal osseointegration. When the primary stability needs to be in the diaphyseal region, the choice of a stem with quadrangular section or longitudinal fins and a short stem is always a priority objective. It is, also, especially necessary to underline the advantages of modular ancillary instruments which facilitate the application of the press-fit concept during revision: a rasp and especially a modular test prosthesis for the selection of a short stem with a "conical reserve". This allows perfect wedging and makes re-wedging possible.

Part II

Preoperative Planning

The preoperative planning is done in **three** steps:

- **First step**: **radiographic analysis of the femur**
  This evaluation should not be limited to an evaluation of bone defects and the presence of difficulties to extract the bone cement. The entire femur should be evaluated, in particular, its morphotype and the presence of osteoporosis.

- **Second step**: **selection of a surgical strategy**
  To choose a surgical strategy is to first determine the femoral approach and, in a revision with a straight femoral stem of press-fit concept, this choice can be imposed (bone defects, curvature of the femur). The zone of the femur that can be used for primary stability, depends on the choice of the femoral approach. It is also at this moment that one can see that the press-fit concept cannot be applied or might be contraindicated.

- **Third step**: **making a preoperative template**
  To visualize the obstacles that could prevent a rigorous application of the press-fit concept and to determine the references that will serve during surgery.

Preliminary Remarks

1. It is necessary to differentiate between the radiological examination whose objective is the choice of a surgical strategy and the radiological examination which allows, in the longer term, to evaluate the results. This distinction is imperative as certain criteria that are important for a smooth surgical procedure do not play a role in the evaluation of results (deviations of the femur or difficulties to excise cement).

2. Reservations must be made with regard to the existing preoperative classifications [10–12]. They are primarily focusing on the presence and the extent of bone defects which are not always easy to evaluate in detail on the preoperative radiographs. Moreover, when the authors evaluate several parameters, the hierarchic order of these criteria is not always clearly established; this is especially true for femoral deviations.

3. In view of the considerable number of faulty X-rays encountered at the time of the revision of a failing femoral prosthesis, it is important to recall that a surgeon must always have several preoperative X-rays at his disposal; at least: a/p view of the pelvis, a/p view of the hip centered on the loose stem and, especially, a radiograph that shows the femur in a/p and lateral view over a sufficient length (approximately 15 cm beyond the distal extremity of the loose implant).

   What to avoid at all cost !
   - Develop a surgical strategy based on a simple a/p radiograph that shows the femur only over a short distance. A femoral curvature in the frontal plane can go unnoticed, which is always dangerous when a straight stem is chosen.
   - Radiographs with a strong reduction coefficient or long distance X-rays because of the increased risk of underestimating bone defects or a femoral deviation.

4. In revision surgery, a ***global evaluation*** of the femoral bone should be made. To do this, four parameters are taken into consideration: the morphotype and the bone defects, but also the difficulties to excise the cement and the degree of osteoporosis. For each parameter a specific classification is established.

However, these four parameters do not all have the same importance. Thus, they are classified in hierarchic order according to the imperatives imposed by the chosen concept (in this case the press-fit). This approach yields Homogenous Radiographic Groups (HRG) that will subsequently serve as a basis for the choice of a strategic option.

P. Le Béguec et al., *Uncemented Femoral Stems for Revision Surgery*,
DOI 10.1007/978-3-319-03614-4_5, © Springer International Publishing Switzerland 2015

5.1 Analysis of Radiographic Parameters

5.1.1 The Morphotype (Fig. 5.1)

Evaluate the femur in the frontal and sagittal plane on X-rays taken on a length of 15 cm beyond the loose implant. Draw the centro-medullary axis on an a/p view. If the axis is lateralized in the metaphyseal region, or, more rarely, medialized, the femur is considered as curved.

Depending on the presence or not of a femoral curvature, there two choices:

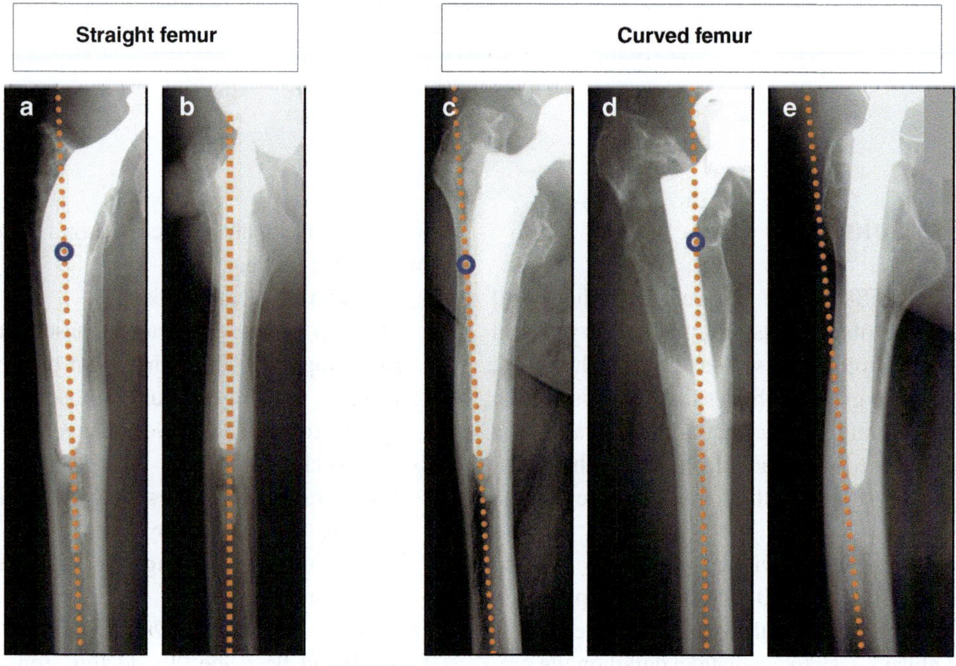

Fig. 5.1 (*Left panel*) Straight femur. Straight femur in the frontal plane (**a**) and slight curvature in the sagittal plane (**b**). (*Right panel*) Curved femur. In the frontal plane: varus curvature (pronounced or not) (**c**) or valgus (**d**). In the sagittal plane: only a global curvature is taken into consideration in the absence of a frontal curvature (**e**)

5.1.1.1 Evaluation of the Morphotype

Except for the classification proposed by Vives and Picault [13], little attention is paid to this evaluation, and most often, we only take note of deviations resulting from a fracture.

In the frontal plane, a femur is straight or curved, the presence of a curvature always constitutes an obstacle.

- Varus deviations are frequent in the case of loose implants, and it is necessary to always take into account curvatures, however slight.
- Valgus deviations are rarer and often the consequence of a fracture, of an osteotomy (Milch) or of a congenital dislocation of the hip.

In the sagittal plane, the femur is often curved, but all curvatures do not constitute an obstacle.

- This is the case for a not very pronounced curvature or for a double sagittal curvature, i.e. diaphyseal curvature with a posterior concavity compensated by a proximal curvature with an anterior cavity, thus resulting in overall straight femur or with little deviation in the sagittal plane.
- On the other hand, a global curvature in the sagittal plane, i.e. a diaphyseal curvature with a posterior cavity which is not compensated by a proximal curvature with an anterior cavity, can constitute an obstacle for the implantation of a straight stem, especially if a long stem is necessary.

5.1.2 Bone Defects (Fig. 5.2)

Evaluate all incidents that could have a weakening effect on the cortices:
- **Granulomas** can sit at a distance and their curettage is difficult by means of an endofemoral approach when they are situated in the isthmic zone
- **Adaptive osseous remodeling**, summarized under the term "stress-shielding", can occur around a cemented or uncemented prosthesis. This is evidenced by decreased bone density and/or reduced thickness of the cortices, which is often the case in patients with osteoporosis.

- **Abrasion of cortices** resulting from an abnormal mobility of the implant/cement couple, and thus entailing mechanical wear of the cortices. In this situation, the extraction of the implant/cement couple is often delicate if the greater trochanter was not opened widely.

Depending on the extent of the bone defects, classify into four stages.

Warning! In the classification below, the zone of the femoral isthmus (zone 4) is usable; if this is not the case, this represents a special case (see table of the Homogenous Radiographic Groups)

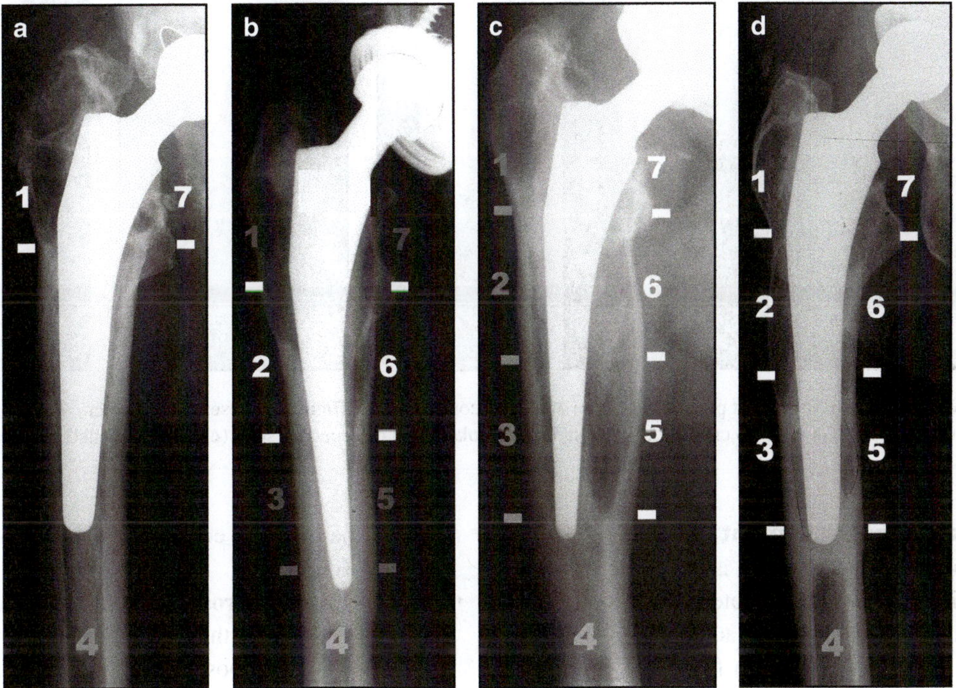

Fig. 5.2 The radiographs that illustrate the above four stages concern only granulomas. **Stage 1**: No defects or localized in zones 1 and/or 7 (**a**). **Stage 2**: Defects in zones 2 and/or 6, possibly in zones 1 and/or 7, but zones 3 and 5 intact (**b**). **Stage 3**: Defects 1 cortex, lateral or medial (zone 3 or 5 is always affected) (**c**) or aggressive granuloma in zone 4. **Stage 4**: Defects 2 cortices: lateral and medial (**d**) or femoral fracture on the stem outside of the zone of the isthmus

5.1.2.1 Evaluation of the 4 Stages
- **Stage 1**: the lesions are strictly localized in the metaphyseal region (zones 1 and/or 7) and there is no femur damage in the metaphyseo-diaphyseal region, zones 2 and/or 6.
- **Stage 2**: lesions in zones 2 and/or 6, often associated with metaphyseal lesions (zones 1 and/or 7). Lesions affecting zone 7 of the metaphyseal region and one other diaphyseal zone are to be included in stage 2 if the defects are localized at this level (example: femoral prosthesis in varus position entailing a bone defect in zone 7 and an erosion of the medial cortex in zone 3).
- **Stage 3**: lesions restricted to one cortex only (mostly the medial cortex), while the other cortex (apart from the greater trochanter) is intact or little affected. In this case, zone 3 or 5 is always concerned as well. Granulomas localized in zone 4, or at a distance, must be classified in stage 3, if they are aggressive.
- **Stage 4**: concerns all lesions that affect two cortices, apart from the greater trochanter. periprosthetic fractures are also classified in stage 4, independent of the quality of the cortices. Fractures in the isthmic zone constitute a particular case.

Nb. Bone lesions due to stress shielding affect normally both cortices and are classified as stage 4 if the bone density is considerably decreased or the cortices thinned.

5.1.3 The Cement (Fig. 5.3)

Implanting an uncemented revision prosthesis requires the complete ablation of the cement in situ. It is thus important that the surgeon has a good understanding of the difficulties that could arise. Evaluate the cement bed as a whole and take into account the quality of the cortices: cement plug and thickness of the cement as well as the position of the distal extremity of the implant (a/p and lateral view).

The patients are classified into two groups, depending on whether difficulties to excise the cement are expected or not.

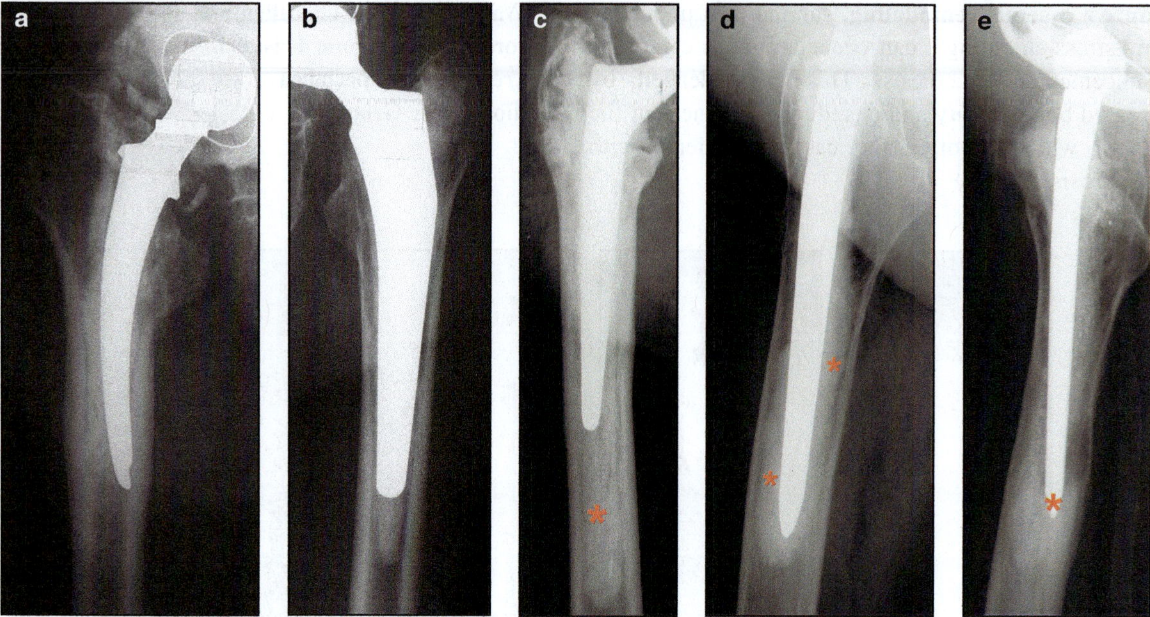

Fig. 5.3 **No difficulties**: No cement plug (**a**) or <3 cm and good cortices (**b**). **Difficulties present**: Plug >3 cm, independent of the quality of the cortices (**c**) or Plug <3 cm or thick cement (sagittal plane) (**d**) or eccentric stem (**e**) **and** weakened cortices

5.1.3.1 Evaluation of the Cement

- **Thickness of the cement bed**. It is advisable to be particularly vigilant in the intermediate zone of the femur if the cement is thick and strongly adheres to a weakened bone. The risk of a via falsa or a fracture is high and a perfect vision of the bone/cement interface is imperative at all times.
- **Cement plug**. Appreciate its length and its adhesion to the surrounding bone. The excision of a cement plug is always difficult, especially if the cortices are weakened. We recall the necessity of complete excision to avoid the risk of eccentric reaming on a remaining cement fragment.
- **At the tip of the prosthesis**. If there is no plug, appreciate the position of the distal extremity of the stem well because eccentric positioning in the a/p or sagittal plane prepares the way for a via falsa. In these circumstances, if no femoral flap was made, a femorotomy in the form of a femoral window is often indicated.

If there is no cement, look for an endosteal bone console which could lead to a via falsa or for a bone plug which is often difficult to pierce

5.1.4 Degree of Osteoporosis (Fig. 5.4)

The degree of osteoporosis is appreciated outside of the zone of stem loosening, in the isthmic region of the femur. It can even be done on the opposite femur. This evaluation is made on the basis of an a/p radiograph. The thickness of the cortices, the geometry of the medullary canal are assessed and the thickness of the cortices or the Cortical Index (**CI**) is measured.

Four stages can be identified:

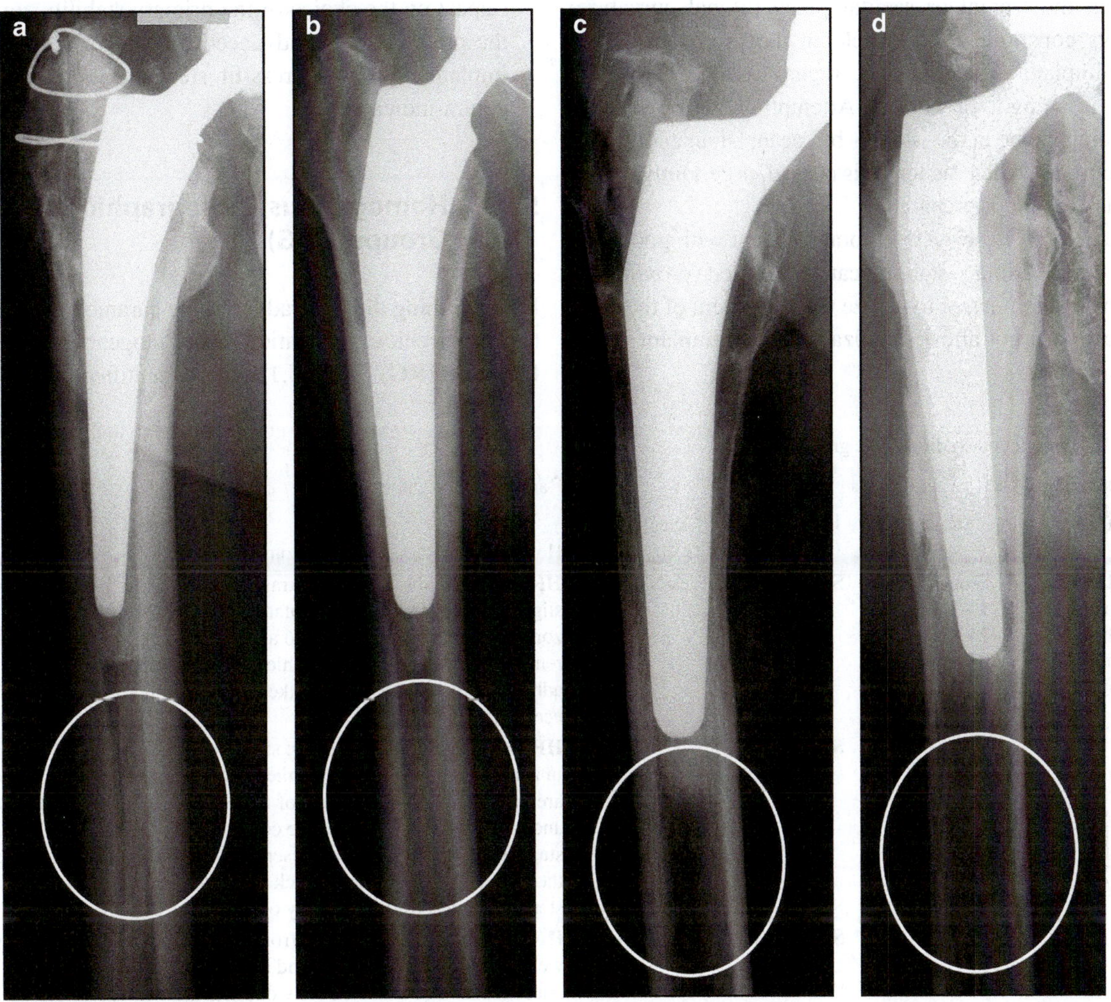

Fig. 5.4 **St. 1 Excellent**: no osteoporosis, thick cortices +, narrow or conical medullary canal + and **CI: =/>0.55 (a)**. **St. 2 Good**: no osteoporosis, thick cortices +/−, conical medullary canal +/− and **CI: 0.45–0.54 (b)**. **St. 3 Average**: osteoporosis +/−, thin cortices +/−, wide medullary canal +/− and **CI: 0.35–0.44 (c)**. **St. 4 Poor**: osteoporosis +, thin cortices +, wide medullary canal + and **CI: =/<0.34 (d)**

5.1.4.1 Evaluation of the Degree of Osteoporosis

- If stages 1 and 4 are usually easy to identify, the same is not true for the intermediate stages 2 and 3. For these cases, the cortical index (CI) is taken into account.
- For stages 2 and 3, take into account also of the geometry of the medullary canal. If medullary canal is cylindrical, the classification is often rated as stage 3. If it is conical, it can be classified as stage 2, even if the cortices are not very thick.
- The notion of a conical medullary canal can correspond to a medullary canal of cylindrical aspect, which, with the help of the reamers, can be reamed to a tapered configuration if the cortices are sufficiently thick. On the other hand, a medullary canal must be considered as cylindrical if it is difficult to make it conical with the reamers because the cortices are too thin.
- Stage 4, corresponding only to a small number of patients, must be identified because it is at this level that the limits of the concepts "fill and fit" or "press-fit" are situated, especially when the choice of a long stem and of a large diameter is indispensable.

5.2 Hierarchic Classification of Radiological Parameters

5.2.1 Primary Parameters

- The morphotype because the presence of a femoral curvature in the frontal or sagittal plane (global curvature) always constitutes an obstacle in the preparation of a bone/implant surface contact, regardless of whether the stem is straight or curved. Attempting to prepare the anchorage zone in the isthmus by means of an endofemoral approach when the femur is curved, is certainly taking the risk of a poor preparation.
- Bone defects, to select a femoral segment with good cortices where primary stability can be ensured (proximal or diaphyseal femur), or to realize that the extent of the bone defects does not allow stabilization of an implant in the isthmic zone.

5.2.2 Secondary Parameters

- Cement excision. This parameter is often taken into consideration when the surgeon hesitates between two different strategic options.
- Osteoporosis. The degree of osteoporosis can have an impact on the choice of the primary stability zone and in the presence of an advanced osteoporosis (stage 4), the implantation of a press-fit stem can be impossible or contra-indicated!

5.3 Homogenous Radiographic Groups (HRG)

By combining the four radiographic parameters according to their hierarchic classification, **six H**omogenous **R**adiographic Groups (**HRG**) (Table 5.1) can be identified.

Table 5.1 Homogenous radiographic groups

Radiographic analysis				Radiographic synthesis
Morphotype (straight or curved)	Osteoporosis (4 stages)	Bone defects (4 stages)	Cement (difficulties)	Homogenous Radiographic Groups (HRG)
Straight femur Frontal plane (1) (1) Sagittal plane: straight femur or slightly curved	**Stages** **1 – Excellent** **2 – Good** **3 – Average**	**Stage 1**	Yes/No	**HRG 1:** Favorable situation: straight femur in the frontal plane and only slightly curved in the sagittal plane. No defects or localized defects in zones 1 and/or 7 (zones 2 and 6 are intact), but possible difficulties to remove bone cement: plug or thick cement in sagittal plane that strongly adheres to the cortices +/– weakened by osteoporosis stage 3 or an eccentric stem
		Stage 2	No / Yes	**HRG 2:** Intermediate situation: straight femur in a/p plane with defects in zones 2 and/or 6 and sometimes in zones 1 and/or 7, but zones 3 or 5 are intact. Careful assessment of the extent of the defects in zones 2 and/or 6; take the quality of the cortices into consideration (osteoporosis stage 3), and especially the presence of possible challenges to remove the cement: cement plug or thick cement (sagittal plane) or eccentric stem with cortices fragilized by osteoporosis stage 3
		Stages 3/4	Yes/No	**HRG 3:** Straight femur in the frontal plane, but defects that entail weakening of 1 or 2 cortices and affect, in all cases, the cortices in zones 3 and/or 5. This is mostly due to a granulomatous disease; more rarely, due to abrasion of one or two cortices because of loosening of bone and cement. If this weakening is due to stress-shielding or to osteoporosis, usually both cortices are affected
				Note: The femoral isthmus can still be used, and if this is not the case (osteoporosis stage 4 or bone defect ++), option 6 is recommended
Curved femur Frontal or sagittal plane (2) (2) Global curvature sagittal plane	**Stages** **1 – Excellent** **2 – Good** **3 – Average**	**Stage 1**	No / Yes	**HRG 4:** Intermediate situation: only slight curvature in a/p plane (1) and no defects. Careful assessment of possible difficulties to excise the cement: peg or thick cement in sagittal plane and strongly adhering to cortices weakened by osteoporosis stage 3 or an eccentric stem. If pronounced curvature in a/p plane or if overall curvature in sagittal plane, see option 5
		Stages 2/3/4	Yes/No	**HRG 5:** Pronounced femoral curvature in the frontal plane or global curvature in the sagittal plane or only slight curvature, but associated with defects stage 2 or more
				Note: If the femur is straight in the a/p plane, only a pronounced curvature in the sagittal plane is taken into consideration (global curvature)
Straight femur or curved	**Isthmic zone destroyed or osteoporosis stage 4**		Yes or No	**HRG 6:** Particular situation characterized by the destruction of the zone of the femoral isthmus (fracture of the femur, iterative loosening of a long stem) or advanced osteoporosis (stage 4) with very thin cortices and a wide and cylindrical medullary canal

The choice of a strategy is only possible after a complete and rigorous analysis of the radiographic parameters which allow *"to base the reasoning on facts and events"* (A.C. Masquelet).

When we choose an uncemented implant with a press-fit concept, ensuring a bone/implant surface contact is a primary objective. *To establish a surgical strategy means to first choose a femoral approach* which allows to access without much difficulty a healthy and rectilinear segment of the femur.

Two options are possible:

- **An endofemoral approach** to ensure, first and foremost, primary stability in the proximal region of the femur, i.e. usually in the metaphyseo-diaphyseal zone.
  NB. A trochanteric osteotomy is similar to an endofemoral approach.

- **A femorotomy** by means of a lateral and pediculated trochantero-diaphyseal flap, if needed, combined with an osteotomy of the medial cortex. In this case, a true press-fit effect can be achieved only in the diaphyseal region of the femur.

Every **H**omogeneous **R**adiographic **G**roup corresponds a strategic option.

P. Le Béguec et al., *Uncemented Femoral Stems for Revision Surgery*,
DOI 10.1007/978-3-319-03614-4_6, © Springer International Publishing Switzerland 2015

6.1   Three Main Options

Every **H**omogeneous **R**adiographic **G**roup corresponds to a strategic option. Options corresponding to **H**omogeneous **R**adiographic **G**roups **1**, **3** and **5** are the three main options which all offer a preferred choice with regard to the femoral approach and a possible alternative choice.

6.1.1   Option 1

HRG 1: **Straight femur in the frontal plane** and not very curved in the sagittal plane. **No defects** or localized defects in zones 1 and/or 7 (zones 2 and 6 are intact), but possible difficulties to remove the bone cement and/or osteoporosis stage 3.

- **An endofemoral approach**, preferred option. Large lateral and posterior opening of the greater trochanter. If necessary, a femoral window can be performed to remove abundant cement in the distal femur (Fig. 6.1)

and/or cement adhering to cortices weakened by an osteoporosis stage 3.

Most often, the press-fit area is situated in the metaphyseo-diaphyseal zone, rarely in the metaphyseal zone. This must be the option of choice in the presence of beginning osteoporosis (stage 3) and, if necessary, bone grafts should be inserted in the endomedullary cavity. In all cases, the selection of a short stem must be the rule (Fig. 6.2).

If proximal fixation is precarious, it is possible to seek additional diaphyseal fixation to achieve a +/− global anchorage of the implant

- **A trochanteric osteotomy** is a possible option when proximal primary stability of the implant is desired (osteoporosis stage 3) and if the greater trochanter is weakened (granulomas) or when it constitutes an obstacle (coxa vara or ATCD osteotomy), or in cases of articular stiffness and/or a subsided implant +.

If a trochanteric osteotomy is envisaged, and if the ablation of cement is difficult, a femoral flap is often preferable (see option 3).

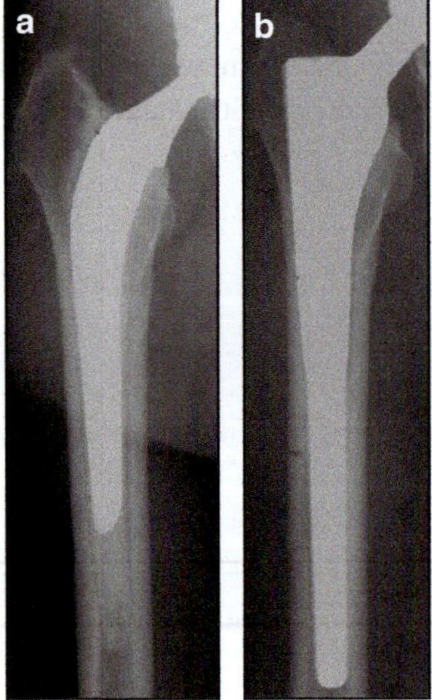

Fig. 6.1 A 66-year-old woman, early loosening of femoral stem. Straight femur and cement plug +, good cortices osteoporosis st.2, CI: 0.50 (**a**). Revision by means of an endofemoral approach to seek proximal stability as a top priority. Femoral window to remove a distal plug of cement. No bone grafts (**b**)

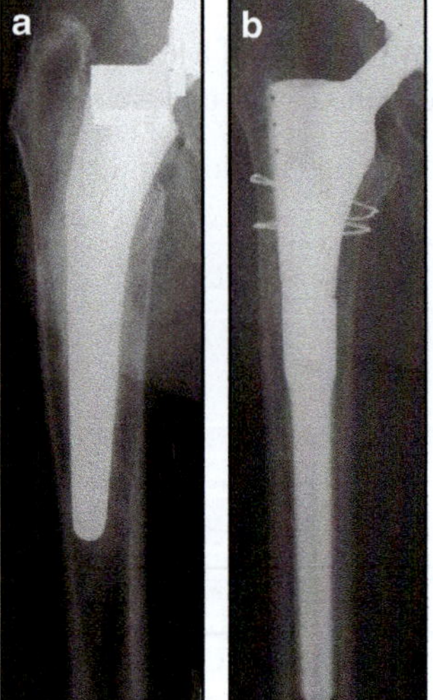

Fig. 6.2 A 71-year-old woman, loosened acetabular cup, granuloma in the medial femoral cortex. Straight femur, no cement plug but osteoporosis st.3, CI: 0.35 (**a**). Revision by means of an endofemoral approach to seek proximal stability as a top priority and to avoid, in such a case, a primary stability only in the diaphyseal region. Cerclage wiring of the proximal femur and intra-medullary cancellous bone grafts (**b**)

6.1.2   Option 3

HRG 3: Straight femur in the frontal plane and only slightly curved in the sagittal plane, **but defects stage 3** (1 cortex) **or stage 4** (2 cortices) and, in both cases, zones 3 and/or 5 are affected. If the isthmic zone is not usable, see option **6**.

- **Trochantero-diaphyseal femoral flap** preferred choice.

  The anchorage zone is in the diaphysis, in the region of the isthmus, and primary stability is ensured over a short distance (3 cm). (A bone/implant contact >5 cm is neither necessary nor desirable). Ensure proximal stabilization of the implant if the cortices are of good quality (Fig. 6.3).

  This maneuver also helps to avoid implantation of a long stem and facilitates secondary proximal osseointegration.

- **An endofemoral approach** is a possible option if the defects are localized and affect only one cortex (with only slight weakening in zone 3 or 5), and if there are no major difficulties to excise the cement. Such a case can be encountered in a situation with osteoporosis stage 3 and/or stress-shielding. In this case, a proximal primary stability is always sought and insertion of an endomedullary bone graft can be necessary. If proximal stability is precarious, seek additional diaphyseal fixation to achieve a +/− global fixation (Fig. 6.4).

If a femoral window is necessary to excise the cement, the option of a femoral flap is often preferable. Remember that a trochanteric osteotomy facilitates proximal fixation

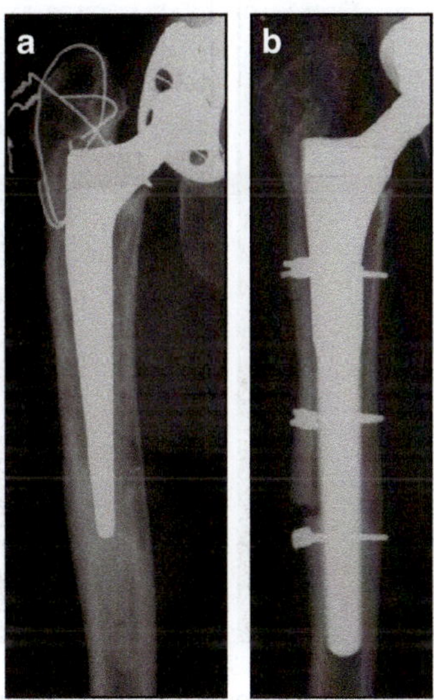

Fig. 6.3 A 63-year-old woman. Cup and femoral stem loosened. Straight femur but medial cortex weakened by granulomas, cement plug +, osteoporosis st.3, CI: 0.44 (**a**). Revision by means of a trochanteric-diaphyseal flap and short diaphyseal stability, no bone grafts (**b**)

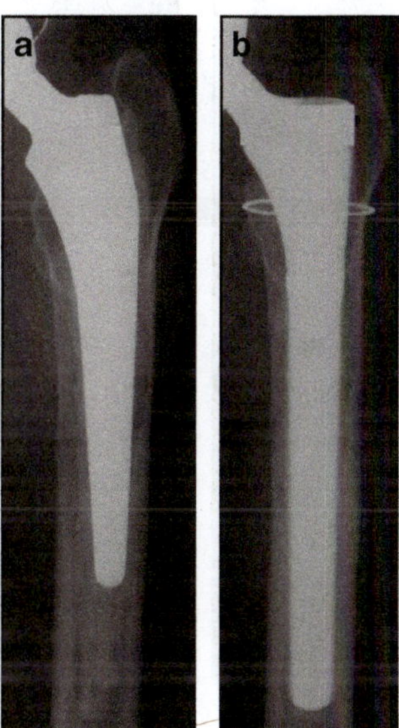

Fig. 6.4 A 69-year-old woman, loose acetabular cup. Femur: granulomas in zones 2 and 6, cement plug +, osteoporosis st.3, CI: 0.36 (**a**). Revision by endofemoral approach to seek +/− global stability and to avoid only diaphyseal primary stability. Cerclage wiring of the proximal femur and intra-medullary adding of HAP granules (**b**)

6.1.3 Option 5

HRG 5: Isolated but pronounced femoral curvature in the frontal plane or global curvature in the sagittal plane; **or** curvature not very pronounced but associated with another obstacle (defects stage 2 or more, or difficulties with the cement). If the isthmic zone is not usable, see option **6**.

- **A femoral flap.** This is the usual option. Seek a short diaphyseal stability in the region of the isthmus. An osteotomy of the medial cortex is associated with a flap to improve (or even ensure) primary stability, provided the cortices are good, while also favoring secondary osseointegration (Fig. 6.5).

- **A trochanteric osteotomy** is a possible option if the curvature is accentuated +/− and defects stage 2 to seek proximal fixation if osteoporosis stage 3 and to avoid an exclusively diaphyseal fixation (Fig. 6.6).

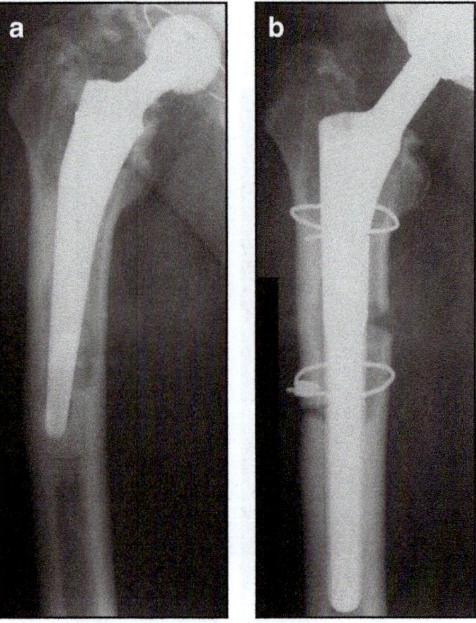

Fig. 6.5 A 58-year-old man, loose femoral stem. Curved femur with medial cortex weakened in zones 5 and 6. No osteoporosis, excellent CI: 0.56 (**a**). Revision with a trochanteric-diaphyseal flap, short diaphyseal stability and osteotomy of the medial cortex, no bone grafts (**b**)

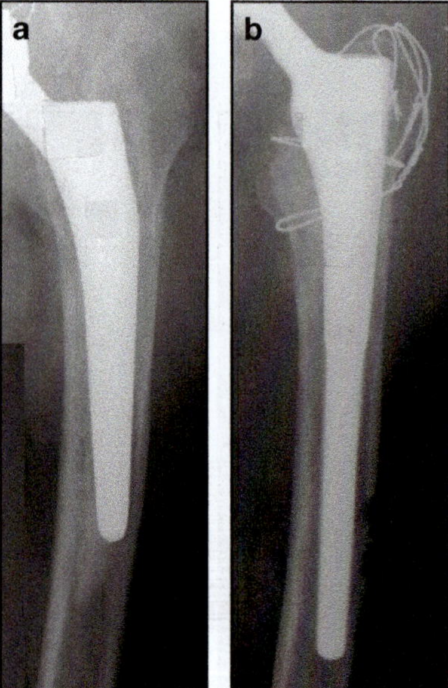

Fig. 6.6 A 71-year-old woman, loose femoral stem. Curved femur with medial cortex +/− weakened in zones 3 and 6 (st.2). Wide medullary canal and CI st.3, average: 0.39 (**a**). Revision by trochanteric osteotomy approach in the only purpose of achieving proximal stability and avoiding diaphyseal stability. Proximal bone graft and femoral window for ablation of the distal cement (**b**)

6.2   Intermediate Options

Options 2 and 4 are intermediate options with two possible choices.

6.2.1   Option 2 (HRG 2)

Defects are localized in zones 2 and/or 6 and sometimes in zones 1 and/or 7, but zones 3 or 5 are intact; take into consideration an osteoporosis stage 3 and whether or not cement removal poses difficulties.
- A femoral flap, if there are difficulties to remove the cement. Favor a short diaphyseal stability (Fig. 6.7).
- An endofemoral approach, if there are no difficulties to remove the cement. If needed, add endomedullary bone tissue or to look for additional diaphyseal stability (Fig. 6.8).

6.2.2   Option 4 (HRG 4)

- Slight curvature of the femur in the a/p plane, and no defects. Take into consideration an osteoporosis stage 3 and whether or not cement removal poses difficulties.
- Often femoral flap, but trochanteric osteotomy possible if proximal stability strongly desirable (osteoporosis stage 3) (see Fig. 6.6).

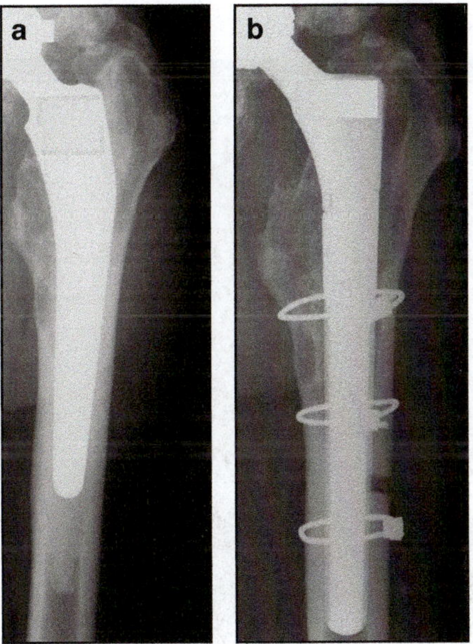

Fig. 6.7 A 70-year-old man, revision of cup. Straight femur with medial cortex weakened by granulomas in zone 6. Cement plug, good CI: 0.48 (**a**). Revision with a trochanteric-diaphyseal flap, short diaphyseal stability and osteotomy of the medial cortex, no bone grafts (**b**)

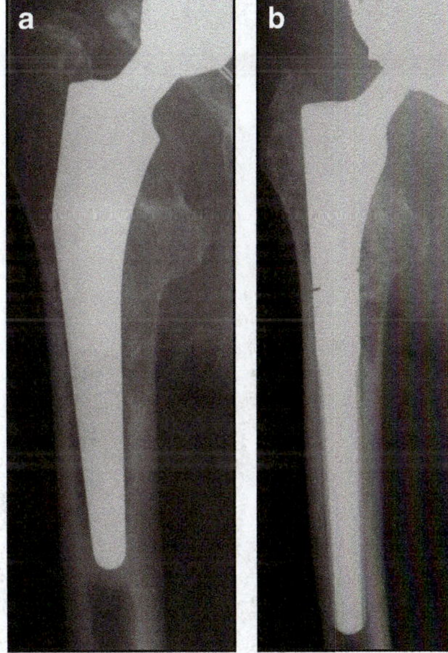

Fig. 6.8 A 84-year-old man, revision of femoral stem. Straight femur with medial cortex weakened by granulomas in zone 6. No cement plug, good CI: 0.51 (**a**). Revision by endofemoral approach and bone grafts, additional, short diaphyseal stability because precarious proximal stability (**b**)

6.3 Option 6 Specific

HRG 6: Destruction of the zone of the femoral isthmus, (fracture of the femur, iterative loosening of a long stem) **or presence of advanced osteoporosis (stage 4)** with very thin cortices and a wide medullary canal.

The *limitations and contra-indications* of the press-fit concept are found in this category.

- Femoral isthmus destroyed: it is recommended to resort to another concept because the press-fit concept is not applicable at the level of the distal third of the femur. In this situation, a self-locking stem finds its elective indication here, especially if the cortices are of satisfactory quality. A technique as proposed by Kerboull [14] is also a possible alternative.
- Advanced osteoporosis (stage 4) with thinned cortices and a wide and cylinder-shaped medullary canal. In this situation it is imperative to look for proximal fixation (Fig. 6.9). If this mode of primary stability is not possible, the press-fit concept is not recommended in these cases because implantation of a long stem with a large diameter in the diaphyseal region often entails serious alteration of the bone stock due to stress shielding. A technique involving massive bone grafting, type Exeter or as proposed by Kerboull, are possible alternatives.

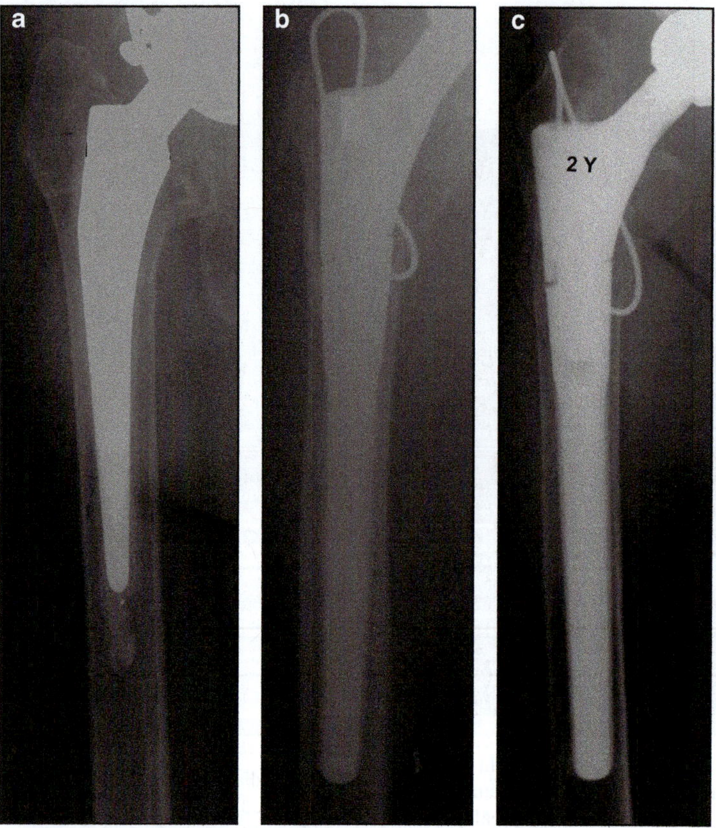

Fig. 6.9 A 64-year-old woman, cup loosened, straight femur, cortices thinned +, wide medullary canal and poor CI <0.34 (**a**). Revision by trochanteric osteotomy to seek proximal stability and avoid diaphyseal fixation (**b**). Result at 2 years: no major modifications of the cortices in the diaphyseal region (**c**)

Table 6.1 Summary of strategic options

Analysis of radiographic parameters				Rx summary	Strategic options		
Morphotype	**Osteoporosis**	**Defects**	**Cement**	**HRG**	**N°**	**Femoral approach**	**Zone of stability**
Straight/curved	4 stages	4 stages	Difficulties				
Straight	Stage 1–3	**Stage 1**	Yes/No	**Group 1** (Favorable)	1	Endofemoral Troch. osteotomy	Proximal Global +/–
		Stage 2	Yes No	**Group 2** (Intermediate)	2	Femoral flap and short diaphyseal fixation **or** proximal on flap Endofemoral or troch. osteotomy and proximal **or** +/– global fixation	
		Stage 3/4 (Intact isthmus)	Yes/No	**Group 3** (Difficulties +)	3	**Femoral flap** Endofemoral or troch. osteotomy	**Short diaphyseal or proximal on flap** Global +/–
Curved	Stage 1–3	**Stage 1**	Yes No	**Group 4** (Intermediate)	4	Femoral flap and short diaphyseal fixation **or** proximal on flap Endofemoral or troch. osteotomy and proximal **or** +/– global fixation	
		Stage 3/4 (Intact isthmus)	Yes/No	**Group 5** (Difficulties +)	5	**Femoral flap** Trochanteric osteotomy	**Short diaphyseal or proximal on flap** Proximal or +/– global
Straight or curved	**Destroyed femoral isthmus**		Yes/No	**Group 6** (Special case)	6	Destroyed isthmus : self-locking stem	
	Stage 4 osteoporosis					Stage 4 osteoporosis: proximal fixation or other concept	

The preoperative template summarizes the entire preoperative reflection.

- Its goal is to visualize the obstacles detected during the radiographic analysis and to determine the key references that will be useful during surgery.
- It is not the objective of the preoperative template to determine the dimensions of the implant. This is always during the intervention with a trial prosthesis.
- The template is done on an a/p radiograph visualizing the femur on a sufficient length (approximately 15–20 cm) beyond the loosened implant to avoid an error of the axis.

7.1 Preoperative Template if Endofemoral Approach

Note: This description is only relevant for the proposed method and refers to a straight uncemented femoral stem.

7.1.1 Draw the Outlines of the Femur and Position the Axes (Fig. 7.1)

- Put the radiograph of the femur in vertical position and draw the outlines of the femur in a/p view, visualizing the zones of bone defects, if any.
- Center the template properly in the diaphyseal region and draw the centro-medullary (CM) axis and that of the center of rotation (CR).

To draw the centro-medullary axis, use the template for a long stem and verify its position at the level of the proximal femur, at the level of the lesser trochanter: in this case it must be +/− centered

It is possible to calculate a difference of length to be corrected, knowing that at this point, it is only a simple indication

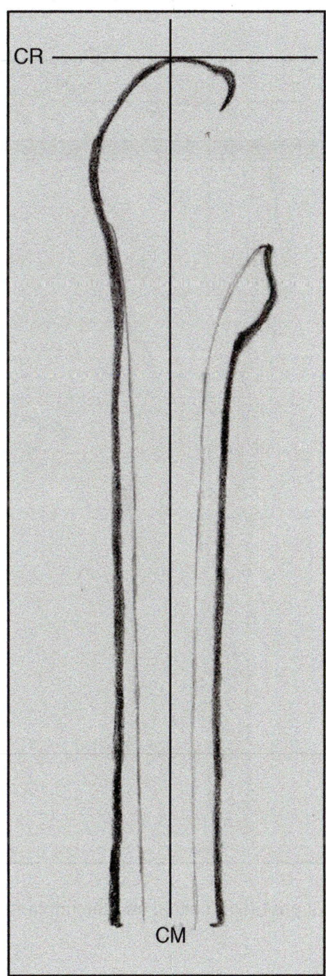

Fig. 7.1 Draw the outlines of the femur and position the axes

P. Le Béguec et al., *Uncemented Femoral Stems for Revision Surgery*,
DOI 10.1007/978-3-319-03614-4_7, © Springer International Publishing Switzerland 2015

7.1.2 Choose the Implant and Visualize the Obstacles (Fig. 7.2)

- Position the template at the correct height on the centro-medullary axis and draw the outlines of the prosthesis.
- Visualize the main bone obstacles. In revision, when the femur is straight and when we choose a straight stem, the obstacles are situated at the tip of the greater trochanter and, in the sagittal plane, at the level of the digital fossa.

Position the tip of the greater trochanter in relation to the lateral cortex

- Visualize the bone defects and the intra-medullary hollow spaces which will need be to filled during surgery.

An intra-medullary bone graft, often in combination with cerclage wiring of the proximal femur, can facilitate the proximal stability of the implant

7.1.3 Determine the Key References (Fig. 7.3)

The depth of penetration (**E**) can be appreciated by the distance between the top of the greater trochanter and the shoulder of the implant.

NB: If the top of the greater trochanter cannot be used, it is possible to refer to the lesser trochanter.

The preoperative selection of the diameter of the implant and of the length of the neck are only indications for the final selection. The final selection is always made during surgery

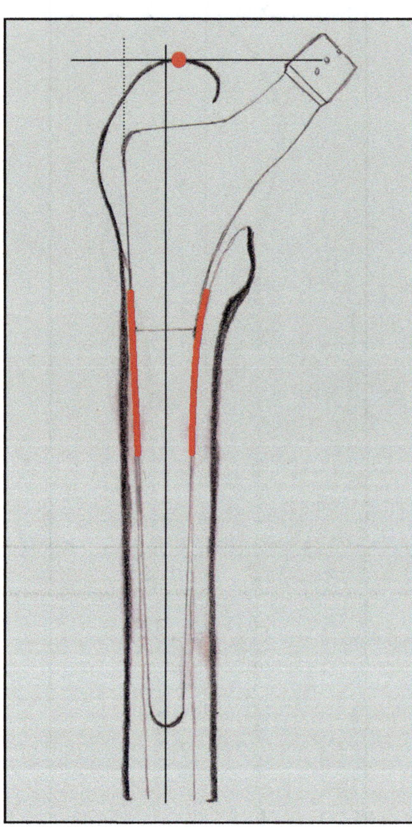

Fig. 7.2 Choose a proximal fixation and the implant

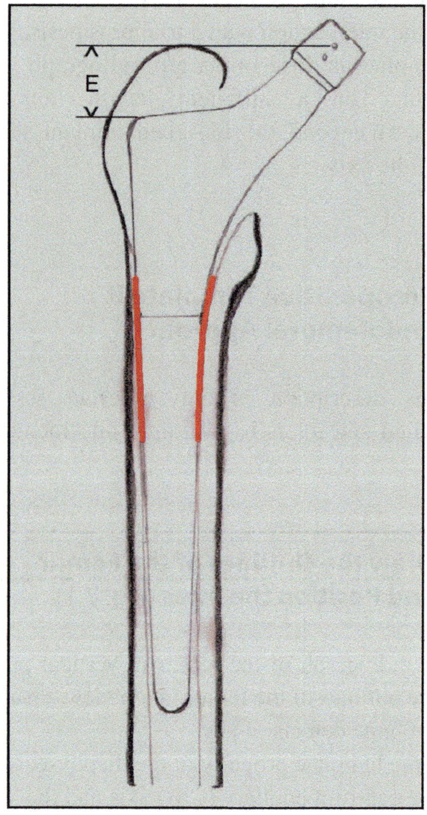

Fig. 7.3 Determine the depth of penetration

7.2 Preoperative Template if Femoral Flap

NB: This description is relevant for a curved femur, but the process is the same when a flap is performed on a straight femur for bone defects or a cement plug.

When a flap is indicated, the preoperative template is done in four stages.

7.2.1 Draw the Outlines of the Femur and Position the Axes (Fig. 7.4)

- Draw the outlines of the femur and visualize the bone defects. **Position the center of rotation of the loose implant and calculate a possible difference of length to be corrected, knowing that this is only a simple indication**
- Trace the axes: centro-medullary (CM) and center of rotation (CR).
  To draw the centro-medullary axis, use the template of a long stem and verify its position at the level of the proximal femur, at the level of the lesser trochanter: in this case it must be +/− lateralized

7.2.2 Determine the Length of the Flap (Fig. 7.5)

- Objective: to access a straight and well corticalized segment of the femur.
- Visualize the distal limit of the flap.
  NB: if there is a curvature in the sagittal plane, the procedure is the same as for a curvature in the frontal plane (perform a lateral flap in combination with an osteotomy of the medial cortex).

In this case, measure the distance between the top of the greater trochanter and the top of the sagittal curvature and transfer this distance on an a/p radiograph.

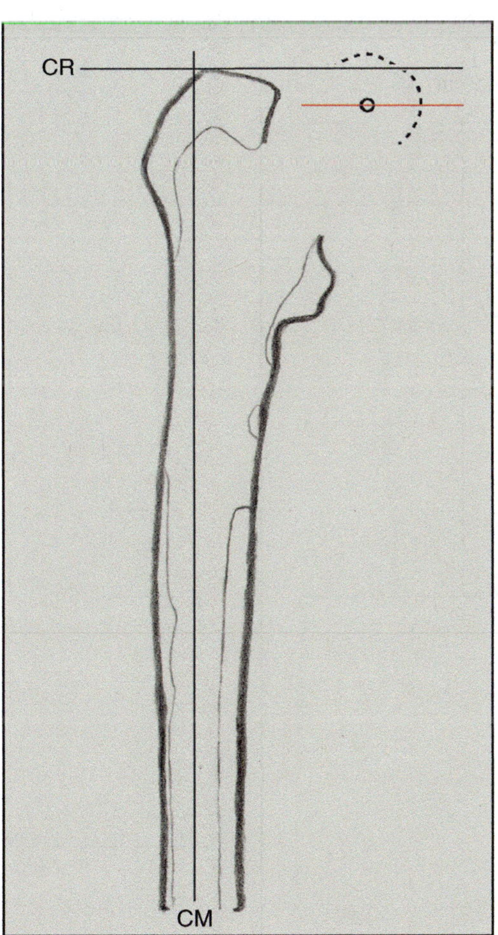

Fig. 7.4 Draw the outlines of the femur and positions the axes. At the level of the proximal femur the CM is lateralized

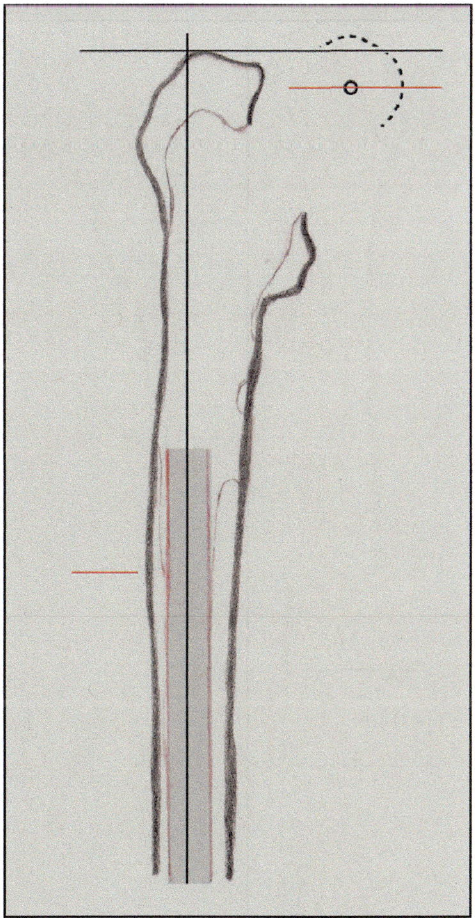

Fig. 7.5 Determine the length of the flap to access a straight segment of the femur

7.2.3   Selection of the Implant (Fig. 7.6)

The final selection is made with the help of a modular test prosthesis.

Reminder. It is impossible to choose the correct implant with a reamer.

- Seek a bone/implant contact of approximately 3 cm in the region of the isthmus with the distal or middle zone of the distal component of the modular trial prosthesis to keep a conical reserve.
- Choose the height of the proximal component of the trial prosthesis to restore the length of the lower limb.
- Determine the level of the medial osteotomy (if the femur is curved) while preserving a chevron.

If you are sure to work on a straight segment of the femur and if, furthermore, we have efficient instruments, the degree of penetration of the trial prosthesis and the definitive implant is the same or easy to correct at the level of L of the neck

7.2.4   Determine the References (Fig. 7.7)

LI   Length of the implant = length of distal component + Height of the proximal component of the trial prosthesis

LV   Median length of the flap: 15–17 cm

E   Degree of penetration = distance shoulder of implant – distal limit of the flap, i.e. length of flap – 2 cm

C   Height of the chevron: 2–3 cm (if a medial corticotomy is performed)

Final implant: the diameter of the implant and the neck length are often selected during surgery

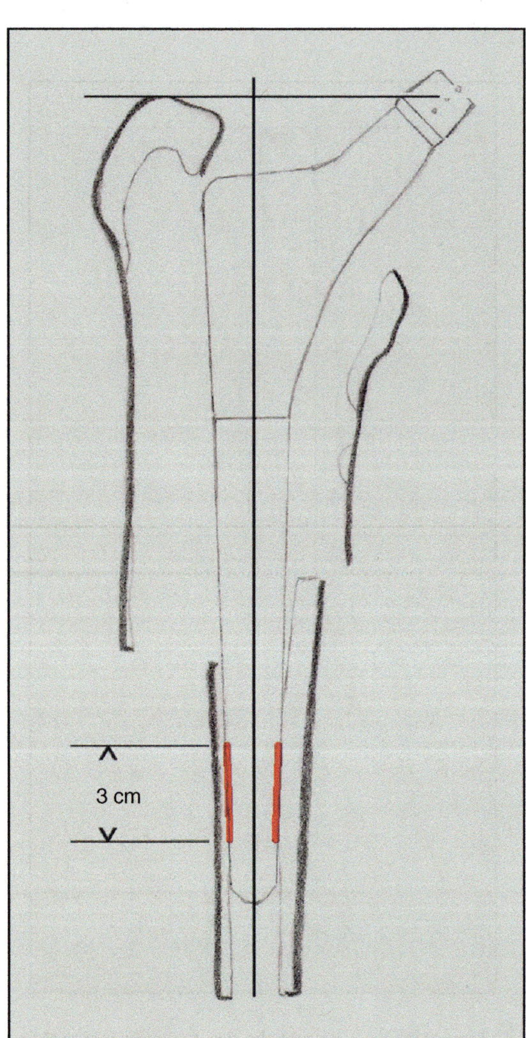

Fig. 7.6 Choose an implant with a short diaphyseal fixation

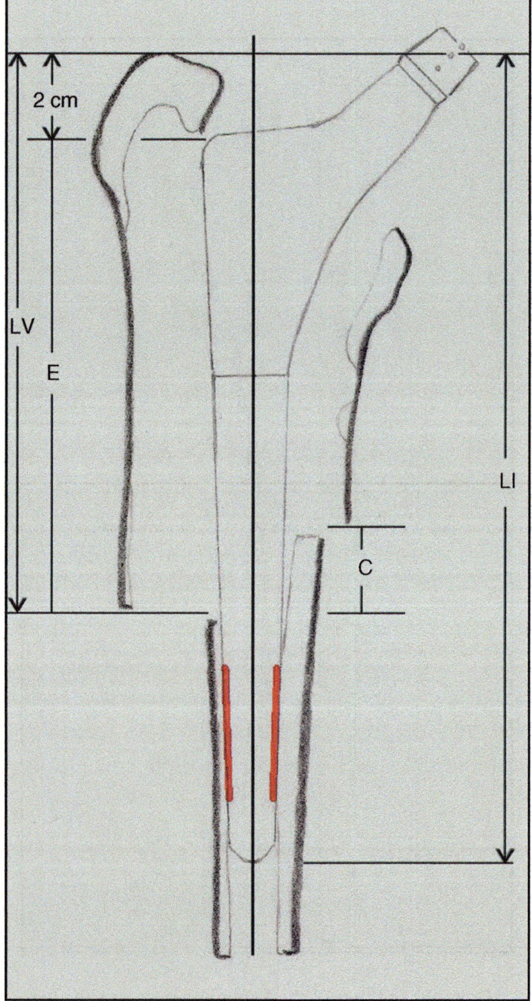

Fig. 7.7 References usable during the surgical operation

Radiographic Analysis

Poor preoperative radiographic analysis is often at the origin of difficulties during the surgical operation and, in the end, the reason for mediocre radiographic results.

It is always dangerous to base the selection of a strategy exclusively or preferentially on a single radiographic parameter because the obstacles the surgeon may have to face during revision surgery are multiple. Thus, when choosing a straight uncemented stem for revision, the surgeon must keep several constants in the mind:

- A femoral curvature in the frontal plane always constitutes an obstacle, even in the absence of bone defects.
- The choice of the zone of primary stability depends on the choice of the femoral approach, i.e. whether or not there are a femoral curvature or bone defects.
- The presence of osteoporosis is to be taken into account at the time of establishing a surgical strategy.
- During revision, it is always necessary to remove all cement. Thus, a good evaluation of the difficulties which can appear in this regard is decisive.

Choice of a Surgical Strategy

During this phase of preoperative reflection, contradictory objectives often have to be conciliated; the most frequent being the necessity of removing obstacles that could hinder the insertion of a straight stem, while at the same time preserving the zone of the femur where primary stability of the implant is possible or desirable.

In a revision case, an endofemoral approach is only envisaged if the femur is not too damaged and if it is straight in the frontal plane. In reality, a trochantero-diaphyseal femoral flap is often indicated: curved femur, damaged cortices or difficulties to excise the cement, and… finally, it is possible to assert that this femoral approach facilitates the revision of a loose femoral prosthesis.

It is also necessary to underline the necessity to seek proximal fixation whenever possible, and to implant a short stem when the primary fixation is sought in the diaphyseal region. These are the two key objectives when choosing an uncemented implant, and particularly the press-fit concept.

Making a Preoperative Template

This third preoperative preparation constitutes a synthesis of the previous two stages.

Reducing the preoperative planning of an intervention to making a preoperative template is an error that is made all too often by a surgeon under pressure. Choosing an implant that can be "inserted" in the endomedullary space such as it appears on a radiograph does not mean choosing a surgical strategy in line with the selected concept of the implant nor with the bone condition of the patient (bone defects and degree of osteoporosis).

Part III

Surgical Technique

Preliminary Remarks

1. Choosing a new implant inevitably involves a learning period, independent of the surgeon's skills. This is actually a good reason for not changing the concept and implant too often!

2. In the case of an uncemented implant, the surgical technique must be particularly rigorous. Technical mistakes often result in an immediate failure.

3. When choosing the press-fit concept, the principles defined by Morscher must always be respected: (1) Obtain a bone/implant surface contact; (2) Ensure perfect wedging of the prosthesis.

4. Bone stock preservation or its regeneration is another objective which is not always easy to reach. Much depends on the design of the implant, on the strategic option and on the surgical technique which must be coherent and mastered.

It is never good to change strategy during surgery.

A femoral osteotomy in the form of a trochanteric- diaphyseal femoral flap, as proposed by Vielpeau et al. [15] and Wagner [2] in the context of a revision, voffers many advantages:

- Easier excision of cement and granulomas while reducing the risks of further damage to the bone stock.
- Reduction of a femoral curvature, mandatory when an uncemented straight or curved stem is chosen.
- Perfect view of the medullar cavity in the isthmic region.

When choosing the press-fit concept, these advantages are decisive for a successful surgery, and to achieve perfect primary stability, which is always situated in the diaphyseal region when a femoral flap has been performed.

preserve the isthmic zone of the femur, the zone for the primary stability of a revision implant.

Indications for a short (# 8 cm) or long flap (# 18–20 cm) are not frequent

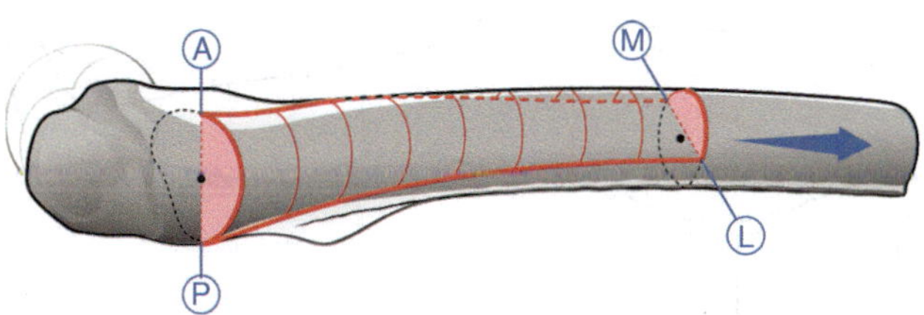

Fig. 8.1 The proximal femur is twisted

8.1 Lateral Trochanteric-Diaphyseal Flap

NB: Description of the surgical technique: prosthesis in place and not dislocated.

8.1.1 General Characteristics

- Both articular approaches – antero-lateral and postero-lateral – are possible, but since we recommend the execution of a lateral trochantero-diaphyseal flap, we prefer a postero-lateral approach.
- The fact that the flap is in a lateral plane in the metaphyseal region and in an antero-lateral plane in the diaphyseal zone (Fig. 8.1), is due to the fact that the proximal femur is twisted. In all cases, the flap is pediculated to the vastus lateralis muscle. The flap is often associated with an osteotomy of the medial cortex.
- The length of the flap, determined before surgery, is about 15±2 cm, the reference point being the top of the greater trochanter. The distal limit of the flap must always

- The flap must be 3–4 cm wide and describe a semicircle in the diaphyseal area (Fig. 8.2). Above all, avoid a flap that is too narrow to reduce a sagittal curvature, and remove any obstacle created by the anterior cortex of the femur during reaming.

  The most frequent error is to make a flap that is too narrow in the diaphyseal region

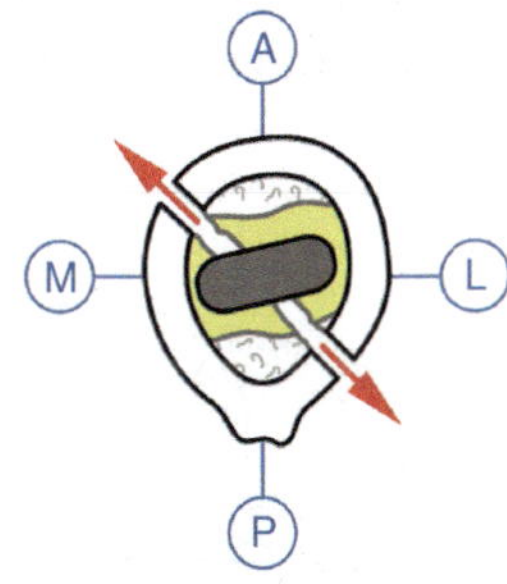

Fig. 8.2 Wide flap in the diaphyseal area

P. Le Béguec et al., *Uncemented Femoral Stems for Revision Surgery*,
DOI 10.1007/978-3-319-03614-4_8, © Springer International Publishing Switzerland 2015

8.1.2 Articular Approach

- The patient is placed in the lateral decubitus position. The pelvis is immobilized dorsally by a sacral support and ventrally by a pubic support (Fig. 8.3).

  Avoid an anterior compression of the femoral blood vessels

  The lower limb is held horizontally by a cushion that can be easily moved so as not to hinder adduction of the hip when the prosthesis is dislocated and the femur exteriorized.

- Posterolateral skin incision centered on the greater trochanter, incision of the facia-lata femoris and the gluteal muscle in the direction of the muscular fibers.

  Soft tissues are retracted with a distractor (Charnley type), which is both stable and rigid.

  Avoid a skin incision too anterior or too posterior

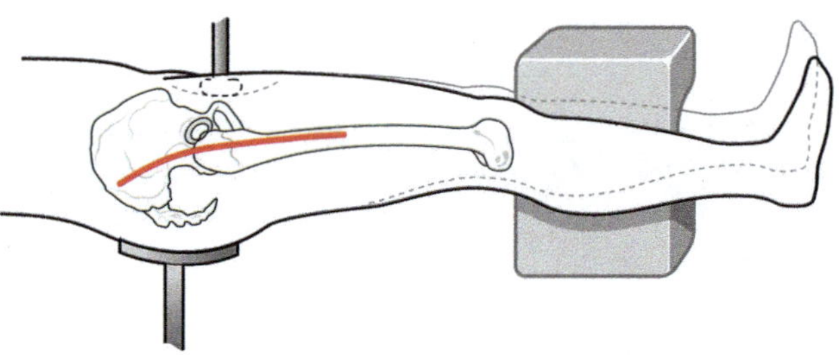

Fig. 8.3 Posterolateral approach: lateral decubitus and skin incision

8.1.3 Exposition of the Femur

- With the help of a spindle, identify the tip of the greater trochanter and, if necessary, enlarge the skin incision. Place the lower limb in slight internal rotation. Section of the quadratus femoris muscle (**1**) and of the aponevrotic extension of the great gluteal muscle (**2**) is performed in most cases.

  Take into account possible calcifications when identifying the tip of the greater trochanter

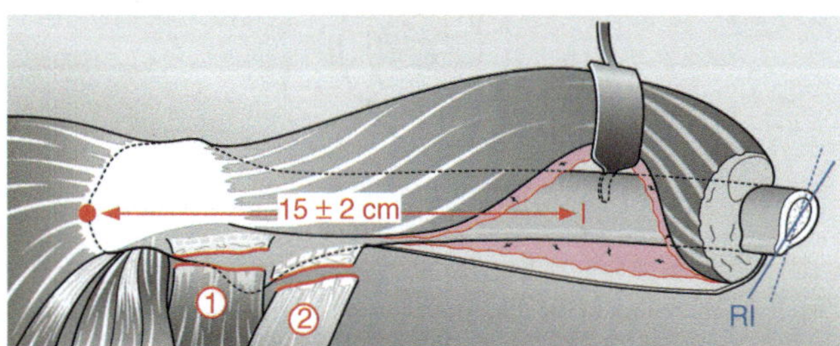

Fig. 8.4 Posterolateral approach: freeing of the vastus lateralis

- Free the vastus lateralis from the intermuscular septum, taking care to cauterize the perforated blood vessels (Fig. 8.4).

  At this moment of the surgery, the short rotators and the posterior capsule are not sectioned

- In the distal region, the vastus lateralis is detached from the femur at a distance corresponding to the length of the flap

  Completely detaching the vastus lateralis from the femur can compromise cortical regeneration or exacerbate secondary necrosis of the femoral flap

- Free the space between the gluteus and vastus lateralis muscles in the proximal region and in front of the hip.

8.1.4 Cortical Osteotomies

- **The distal cut** is perpendicular to the diaphyseal axis, 3–4 cm wide and limited by two drill holes of 4.5 mm.

  Two drill holes to avoid extension of the anterior and posterior cuts beyond the distal cut osteotomy (can trigger a secondary fracture)

- **The posterior cut** is slightly anterior to the external bifurcation of the linea aspera and is curved in the proximal region to protect the posterior insertions of the gluteus medius muscle (Fig. 8.5).

  The posterior and distal cuts are performed with an oscillating saw

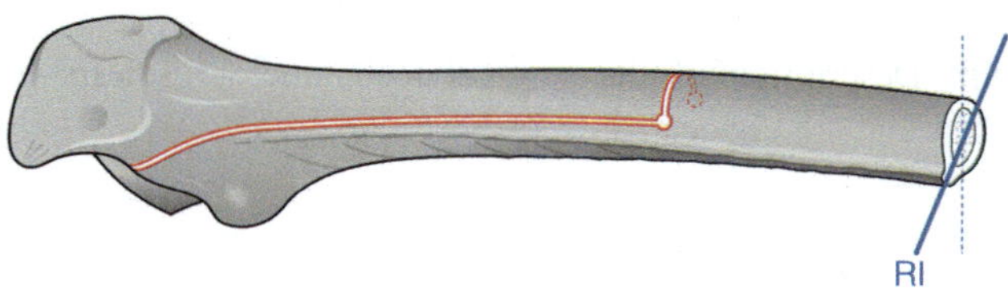

Fig. 8.5 Distal and posterior cuts of the flap

- **The anterior cut** is performed in two steps.
  - Initiate the anterior cut at both extremities: distally with an oscillating saw after performing the transverse cut, and proximally with the help of a bone chisel (Fig. 8.6a).

    If ATCD anterior approach: preliminary excision of fibrous tissues between the gluteus and vastus lateralis

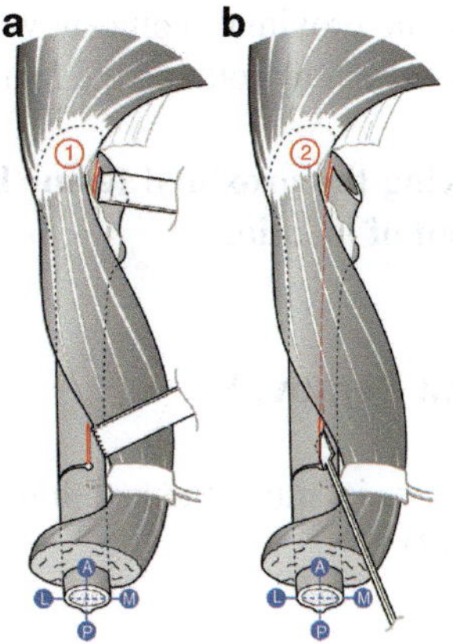

Fig. 8.6   Initiate the anterior cut (1) and finalize with narrow chisel (2)

– Finalize the anterior osteotomy with the help of a narrow chisel which is inserted into the line previously initiated in the distal zone and extend it to the front of the femur, under the vastus lateralis (Fig. 8.6b).

Carefully check that the distal osteotomy in the angles is complete

8.1.5   Freeing the Flap

At this point of the surgery, the flap cannot be mobilized yet. Before this is attempted, all adhering fibers have to be detached: cement and intra-articular.

8.1.5.1 Cement Adherences

- In the distal region, fracture the cement with a bone chisel to spontaneously free the distal part of the flap (Fig. 8.7).

If this does not work, verify if the anterior cortical osteotomy is complete

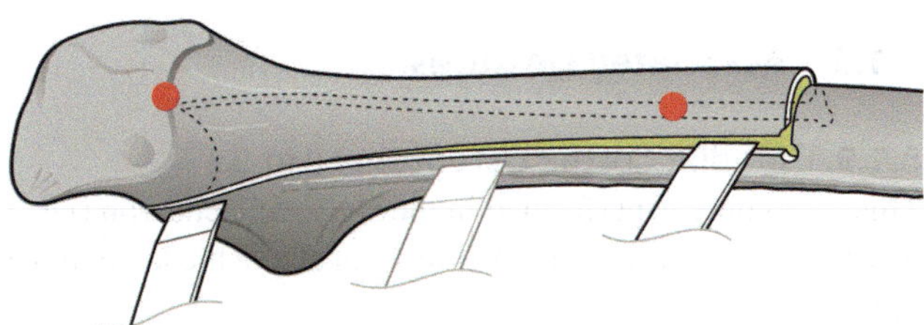

Fig. 8.7   Free the distal part of the flap

- When the distal part of the flap is detached, move towards the intermediary and proximal zones of the femur to fracture the cement which is often abundant at the level of the greater trochanter (Fig. 8.8).

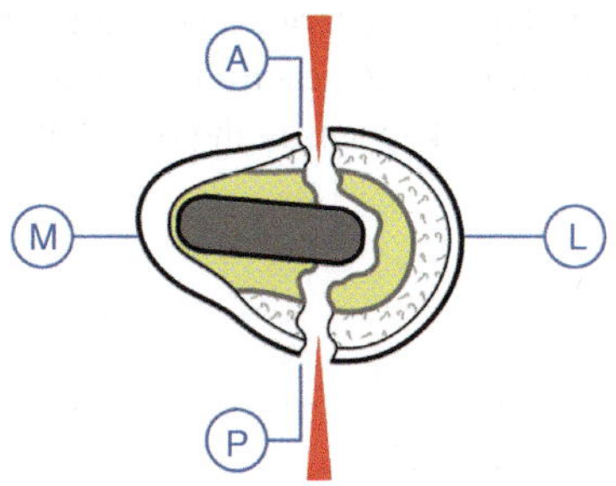

Fig. 8.8   Fracture the cement at the level of the proximal zone

8.1.5.2 Fibrous Attachments to the Intra-articular Cavity (Fig. 8.9)

- Elevate the flap using forceps with points at the level of the greater trochanter (**1**)
- Cut the tendons of the pyramidal, the external rotators and the posterior capsule close to the bone (**2**)

Preserve the external rotators and the posterior capsule for the articular closure

- Free the adhering fibers under the glutei muscles and the greater trochanter (**3**)

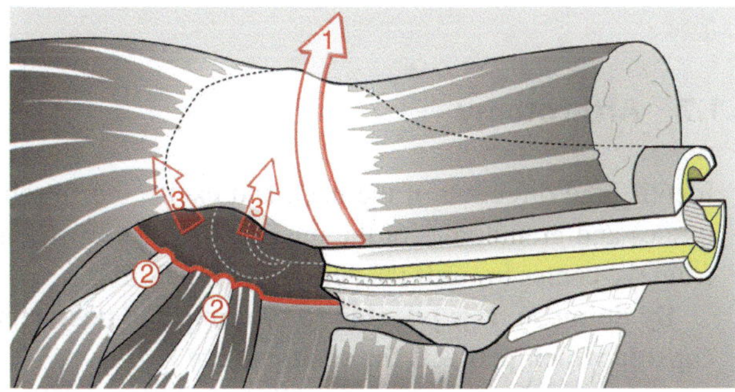

Fig. 8.9   Free the intra-articular cavity

8.1.6 Turning the Flap

- Once freed from all its attachments, the flap is carefully turned around its ventral hinge (Fig. 8.10).

  NB: If turning the flap proves difficult, the cause is often an incomplete anterior osteotomy. In that case, repeat the ventral tilting gesture to complete the anterior cut. This generally happens in the right "place".

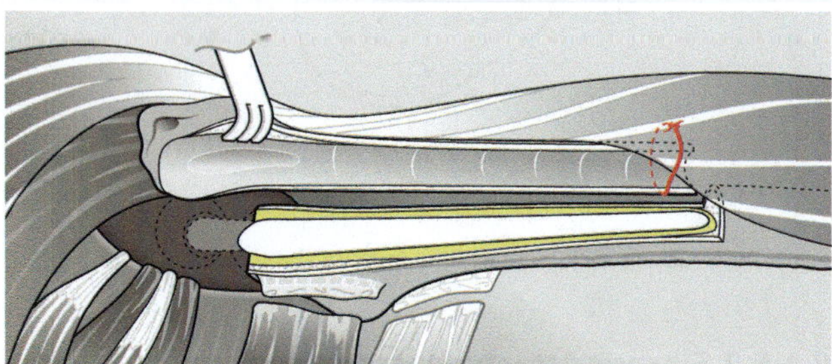

Fig. 8.10 Free the intra-articlular cavity before turning the flap

- Excision of the cement and false membranes; curettage of geodes and granulomas.

  In certain cases, the greater trochanter must be remodeled and the ablation of the cement at this level is sometimes laborious
- To avoid avulsion of the vastus lateralis muscle from the flap, tie together the distal extremity of the flap and the vastus lateralis muscle by means of a transmuscular stitch.

8.1.7 Arthrotomy

- Identify the direction of the neck and excise the fibrous tissues and granulomas of the medullary cavity, working from the center towards the periphery (Fig. 8.11).

  By doing so, it is possible to preserve the posterior capsule which protects the sciatic nerve

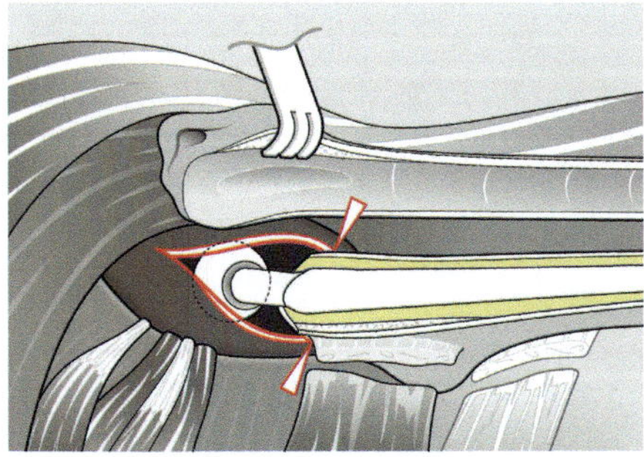

Fig. 8.11 Identify direction of the neck and arthrotomy

- Begin freeing the proximal femur by working closely to the cortical bone and by rotating the femur internally and externally.

  Begin freeing the proximal femur before performing an attempt of luxation

8.1.8 Implant Removal

- Remove the stem in situ if the length of the flap is sufficient (Fig. 8.12).

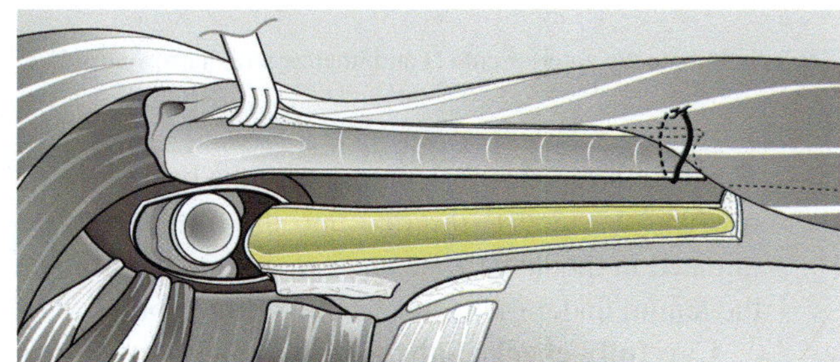

Fig. 8.12 Remove the stem and exteriorization of the femur

- When luxation is required, apply traction on the neck and make a careful combined maneuver of flexion, adduction and internal rotation.

  Remember that the medial cortex of the femur is not fully freed at this stage of the operation
- Finish the proximal detachment to obtain a good exteriorization of the femur.

  A complete exteriorization of the femur is always indispensable

  NB: For the ablation of the cement, see paragraph 9.2 and 10.3, and for putting back the flap back into place, see paragraph 9.6.

8.1.9 Associated Gestures

8.1.9.1 Medial Cortex Osteotomy (Fig. 8.13)

This osteotomy is performed in the shape of a chevron (i.e. a reversed "V") approximately 3 to 4 cm above the lower edge of the flap.

Perform an osteotomy of the medial cortex to restore the contact between bone and implant in cases presenting a varus and/or a sagittal curvature.

Objectives: optimize primary stability and create favorable conditions for secondary stability

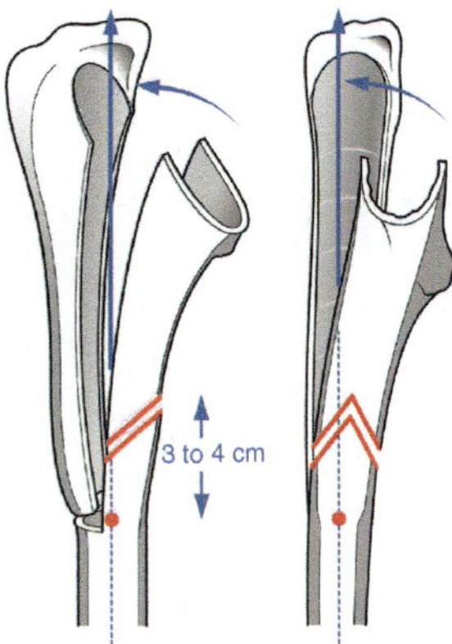

Fig. 8.13 Medial osteotomy

NB: In the presence of a pronounced sagittal curvature, a lateral flap is not always enough to bypass obstacles when implanting a straight stem. An osteotomy of the medial cortex can become necessary, especially if a long stem is used.

8.1.9.2 Cerclage Wiring of the Femur

To avoid or repair a fracture or a crack in the diaphyseal region (Fig. 8.14).

This incident can easily be prevented if the distal cut of the flap is limited by two drill holes of 4.5 mm

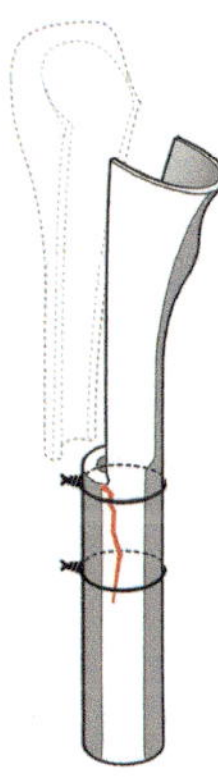

Fig. 8.14 Cerclage wiring if diaphyseal fracture

8.1.9.3 Osteotomy of the Linea Aspera

Systematically recommended by Vives and Picault [13], this osteotomy is only performed when there is distinct shortening of the lower limb and a tight hip. Freeing the linea aspera facilitates the lengthening of the lower limb and the reduction of the prosthesis.

8.2 Technical Alternatives

8.2.1 Anterior Flap

8.2.1.1 Anterolateral Approach (Fig. 8.15)

- Patient in dorsal decubitus position, skin incision centered on the greater trochanter.
- Incision through the gluteus medius and vastus lateralis muscles.

It is difficult to reduce a pronounced femoral curvature in the frontal plane with this technique

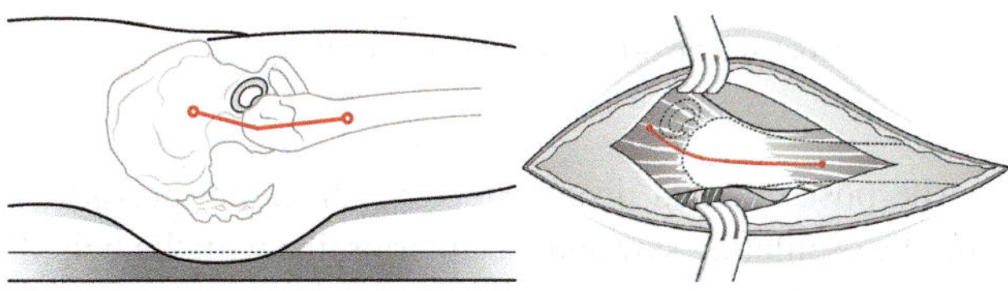

Fig. 8.15 Dorsal decubitus and transmuscular incision

8.2.2 Flap After Luxation and Removal of the Prosthesis

It is possible to perform a flap after luxation and removal of the prosthesis.

Osteotomy of the cortices with an oscillating saw through the medullary canal from the lateral cortex towards the medial cortex, after performing the distal cut (Fig. 8.16).

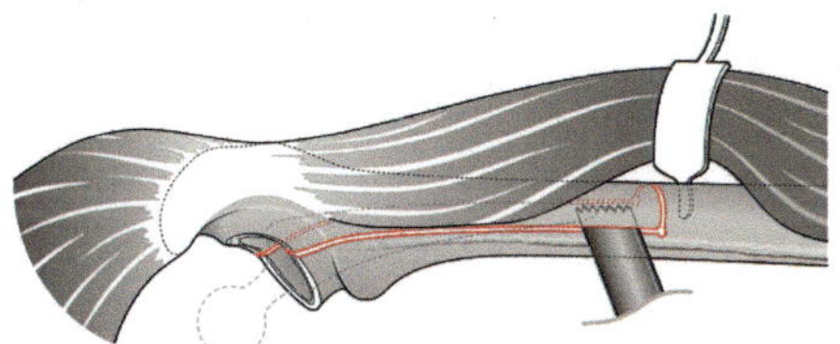

Fig. 8.16 Flap after luxation and removal of the prosthesis

This rather attractive technique implies a luxation of the hip without risking a fracture and is reserved for hips with good articular flexibility and surgeons who have experience with this procedure.

Performing a flap with the same technique, by passing the oscillating saw over the shoulder of the implanted prosthesis from the lateral to the medial cortex, is not advisable because the risks associated with a flap that is too narrow in the diaphyseal region are important

8.2.3 Enlarged Trochanteric Osteotomy

In this case, the muscular fibers of the vastus lateralis are removed, preserving the attachments of the muscle at the base of the greater trochanter (Fig. 8.17).

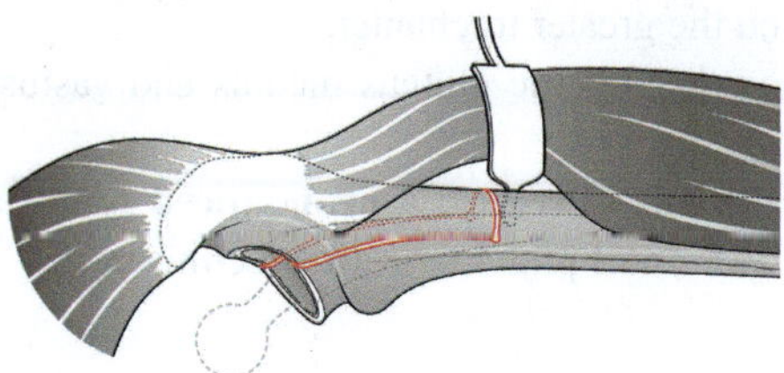

Fig. 8.17 Trochanteric osteotomy enlarged or short flap

The posterior and distal osteotomy lines are performed with the oscillating saw and the anterior line with the help of a bone chisel. The flap is turned ventrally.

This femoral approach can be performed with the prosthesis in place.

This femoral approach can be compared to a short flap (# 8 cm). Its indications are not very frequent (stocky patient or femoral dysplasia)

Femoral Flap and Diaphyseal Primary Stability

In revision surgery, performing a femorotomy in the form of a trochantero-diaphyseal femoral flap is a good way to avoid intra-operative incidents and to ensure a true press-fit effect. In such cases, the press-fit is always situated in the diaphyseal region.

- Both articular approaches – anterolateral or posterolateral – are possible. Yet, as much as we recommend a lateral flap, a posterolateral access is preferable.
- It is in all cases a pedicle flap with the vastus lateralis muscle, in combination with an osteotomy of the medial cortex, if necessary, during or at the end of the surgery.
- Make good use of the reamer for the preparation of the anchorage zone and of the modularity of the trial prosthesis to determine the final prosthesis.
- Whenever possible, implant a short stem with an implant/bone contact over a distance of approximately 3 cm.

9.1 Making a Trochantero-Diaphyseal Femoral Flap

Note: Femoral flap: see Chap. 1 for a detailed description of the operative technique

The patient is placed in a decubitus lateral position, posterolateral skin incision centered on the greater trochanter. Lateral pedicle flap with the vastus lateralis of an average length of 15 ± 2 cm. Always preserve the femoral isthmus, which is the zone of primary stability.

Avoid a flap that is too narrow in the diaphyseal region or a flap that is too long with the sole purpose of removing a cement plug

1. **Prosthesis not dislocated and stem in place**.
- Posterior and distal cuts are done with a saw and the anterior cut with a bone chisel that is inserted under the vastus lateralis muscle.
- Before any attempt of turning it, free the flap from its ties: cement in the medullary cavity (greater trochanter in particular) and adhering fibers in the articular cavity (Fig. 9.1).

If necessary, make gentle lever and ventral rocking movements to complete the anterior osteotomy line which is generally made in the right "place" if the anterior osteotomy was accurately started on both ends.

An incomplete anterior osteotomy is often at the origin of difficulties in turning the flap

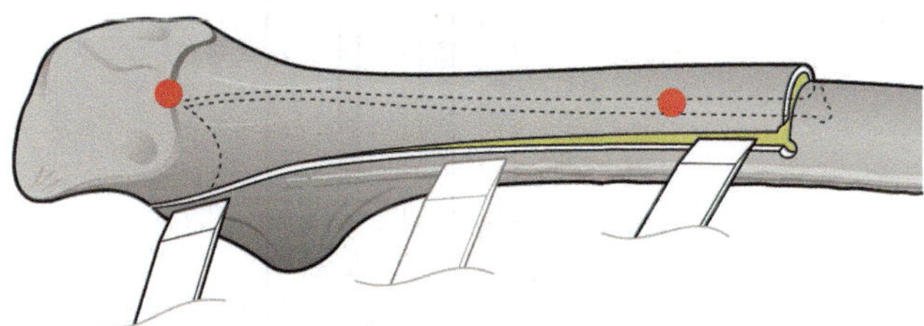

Fig. 9.1 Freeing the flap

2. **After dislocation and the removal of the implant**.
The osteotomies of the cortex are done with a saw from the lateral to the medial cortex and through the medullary cavity after performing the distal cut of the flap.

It is preferable to avoid this technique if the hip is stiff and the cortices weakened

P. Le Béguec et al., *Uncemented Femoral Stems for Revision Surgery*,
DOI 10.1007/978-3-319-03614-4_9, © Springer International Publishing Switzerland 2015

9.2 Cement Removal

Before excising the cement, ensure a perfect exteriorization of the proximal femur after freeing it from its fibrous and capsular attachments (in particular at the medial cortex) and finish cleaning the articular cavity of the acetabulum.

- **The excision of the cement at the level of the flap** and the intermediate zone of the femur (medial cortex) is not a problem as long as you have a good vision of the bone/cement interface, which requires extensive rinsing. Careful curettage of the geodes and granulomas.

  Avoid weakening the greater trochanter too much.

- The excision of a cement plug is made only after complete excision of the intermediate cement. At first, the plug is pierced with a 6 mm diameter drill, while ensuring that it is well centered (Fig. 9.2a). Make sure that you create no via falsa, enlarge the opening to about 11 mm to be able to use a wide cement extractor (Fig. 9.2b).

  If the cortices are weakened (osteoporosis), it is wise to apply a cerclage wiring before the removal of a cement plug

  Complete excision of the cement to avoid eccentric reaming

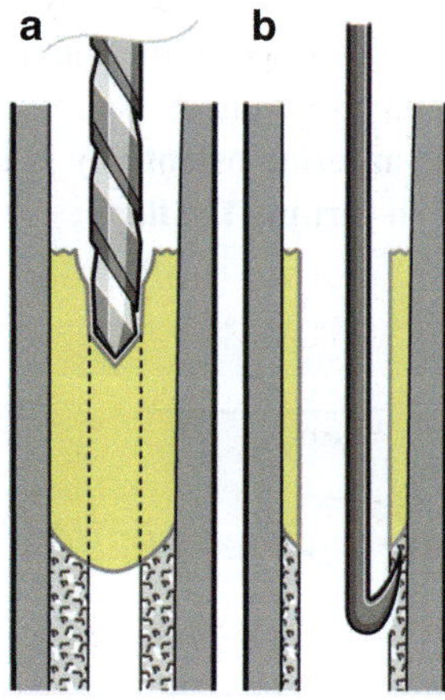

Fig. 9.2 Excision cement plug: pierce the plug (**a**) and excision of the cement with an extractor (**b**)

9.3 Preparation of the Femur

When a femoral flap has been chosen, the preparation of the femur and the choice of the implant are always carried out separately. *The preparation of the femur is performed exclusively with reamers.*

The rasp effect of a trial prosthesis is useless in this situation

9.3.1 Calibrate the Femur and Verify the Axis in the Sagittal Plane

- Eliminate the narrowing zone at the tip of the removed prosthesis with a cylindrical reamer. Calibrate the medullary canal without increasing its diameter, except for when it is narrow (a minimum diameter of 12 or 13 mm is required) (Fig. 9.3).

  Note the proximal diameter of the medullary canal (at the level of the distal cut of the flap)

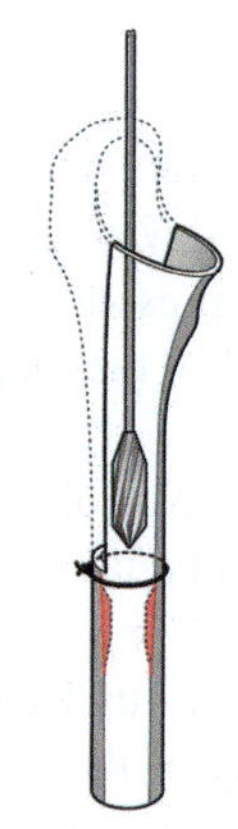

Fig. 9.3 Calibrate the femur

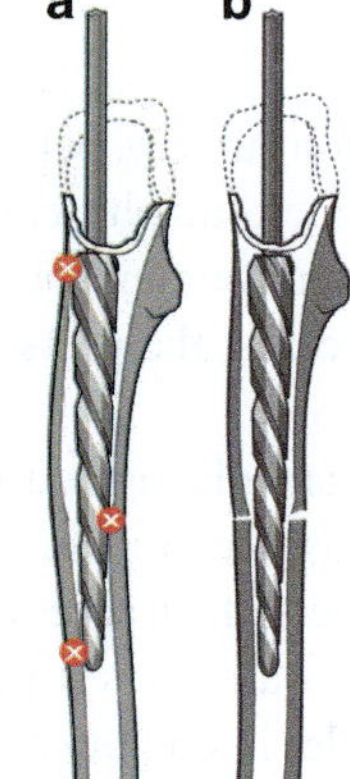

Fig. 9.4 When the anterior cortex is an obstacle (**a**), perform an osteotomy of the medical cortex (**b**)

- Ensure that the anterior cortex is not an obstacle for the progression of the reamer in the axis of the femoral diaphysis (pronounced sagittal curvature) (Fig. 9.4a). To do this, use a long tapered reamer with a diameter that is smaller than that of the medullary canal.

  If the anterior cortex of the femur constitutes an obstacle, it is preferable at this moment of the surgery, to perform an osteotomy of the medial cortex, especially if it is weakened (Fig. 9.4b)

9.3.2 Reaming of the Femur (Preparation of the Anchorage Zone)

The only role of a reamer is *to give the medullary cavity a tapered configuration over a short distance* (3–4 cm) in the diaphyseal zone. Reaming is only started when we are sure to work in a rectilinear segment of the femur.

Reminder: it is impossible to reduce a femoral curvature with a reamer!

1. Choose the diameter of the reamer according to the first indication given by the cylindrical reamer during the calibration of the femur. Start reaming by *using only the distal part of the reamer* (Fig. 9.5).

   If the reamer sinks too far down, increase the diameter; if, on the contrary, it cannot be inserted enough, reduce the diameter.

   During reaming use a clamp for the control of torsional forces

   Reaming with the help of a motor is possible if the cortices are thick; if they are weakened, reaming should be done manually

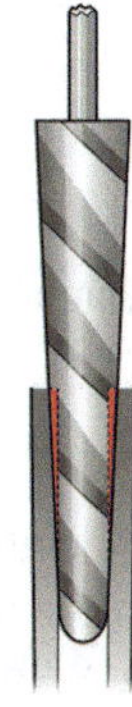
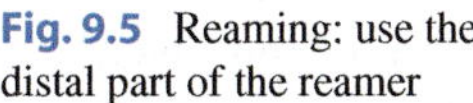

Fig. 9.5 Reaming: use the distal part of the reamer

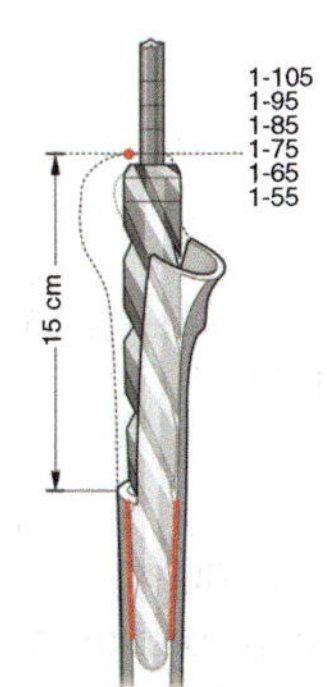

Fig. 9.6 Determine the degree of penetration of the reamer and the references of the trial prosthesis

2. With a sterile ruler, the tip of the greater trochanter is placed on the handle of the reamer at a distance corresponding to the length of the flap, taking the distal cut of the flap as a reference (Fig. 9.6).
   - The tip of the greater trochanter must be in zone 1 (short distal component of 140 mm length) and enable the use of a proximal component of average heigth (65 or 75 mm). This makes it possible to keep a margin of maneuver when choosing the definitive implant.

   It is always preferable to avoid a proximal component of a 95 or 105 mm height

   Example: for a flap of 15 cm length, the tip of the greater trochanter is at the 1–75 mark (Fig. 9.6). This reference corresponds to an implant composed of a distal part of 140 mm length (number 1), coupled with a proximal part of 75 mm height.
   - More rarely, the tip of the greater trochanter is situated in zone 2, which corresponds to a distal part of 200 mm length (rangy patient or long flap).

   When a distal part of 260 mm length is necessary (tip of the greater trochanter in zone 3), it is often preferable to choose a self-locking stem

9.4   Selection of the Implant

At this point of the surgery, *it is necessary to have a modular trial prosthesis* and an exact perception of the usable tapered zone of the trial implant.

Reminder: **it is impossible to choose the right implant with a reamer**
- Assembly of the two components of the trial prosthesis according to the references indicated on the reamer.
- Insertion by means of light blows on the hammer and avoid a forcible impaction to avoid a risk of jamming the stem. Assess the degree of penetration by measuring the distance between the shoulder of the trial prosthesis and the distal end of the flap. This distance must correspond to the length of the flap – 2 cm (Fig. 9.7).

After this step, there are two possibilities:
1. **Presence of a conical reserve**, i.e. primary stability is achieved in the distal or medial portion of the tapered area of the inserted trial prosthesis (Fig. 9.7). This is usually the case if the preparation of the anchorage zone has been done with the distal part of the reamer.

   Trial reduction; if the hip is stable and equal length of the two lower limbs restored, the choice is good.

   To assess the conical reserve, we can take the distal end of the flap as a reference: the proximal line delimiting the usable tapered portion of the trial prosthesis is clearly situated above the distal cut of the flap

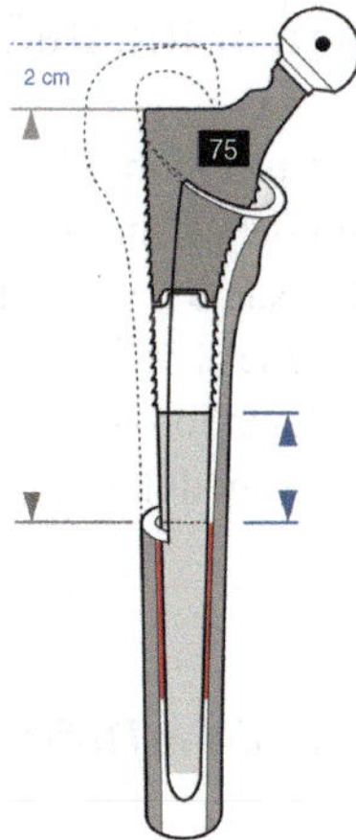

Fig. 9.7 Preserve a conical reserve to ensure a perfect wedging

2. **There is no conical reserve**, i. e. primary stability is achieved in the proximal part of the tapered area.
   - If this is the case with a short distal part (L.140 mm), increase the implant diameter. In this case, additional reaming may be necessary.

- If this occurs with a distal part of 200 mm (Fig. 9.8a): choose a short distal part (L.140 mm) with a diameter +2 mm. This ensures the same filling of the canal while preserving a conical reserve and without lengthening the lower limb (Fig. 9.8b).

There is rarely no conical reserve if the reaming of the femur was done according to the aforementioned rules

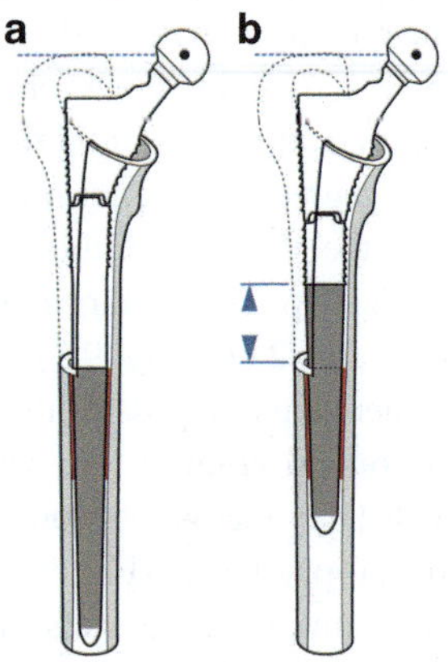

Fig. 9.8 Augment the diameter of the implant (**a**) to keep a conical reserve (**b**)

- Trial reduction, and, if necessary, change the height of the proximal part of the trial prosthesis.

NB: If difficulties during reduction arise, see paragraph 9.7.

9.5 Implantation of the Definitive Stem

- If the definitive stem is a monobloc type, implantation is made in one step, knowing that trial and definitive prosthesis stabilize at the same level if the preparation of the femur (reaming) and the choice of the implant were carefully done. (For implantation in one step, see page 105).
- If the definitive stem is modular, implantation in two steps is possible.

9.5.1 Implantation of the Definitive Distal Part

- Assembly of the temporary proximal part (same height as the trial proximal part) on the definitive distal part. The antetorsion is adjusted in neutral position (Fig. 9.9a).
- Manually introduce the implant with the desired antetorsion in the medullary cavity.
  Do not correct antetorsion during the impaction
- Impaction is done with gentle hammering and while constantly checking the progression of the implant with a sterile ruler. When the progression stops, wait a few seconds and check again to ensure that the progression is finished (cortical sound).

The wedging of the implant is done over a distance of 2–4 cm after manual introduction of the implant in the medullary cavity

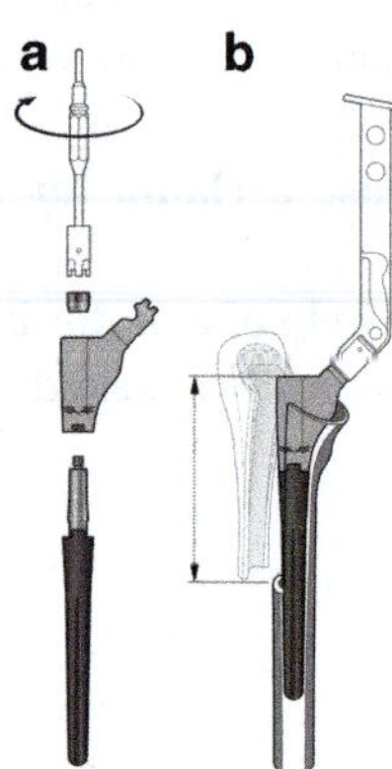

Fig. 9.9 Temporary proximal part (**a**) for implantation of definitive distal part (**b**)

Control the degree of penetration, choose the height of the definitive proximal part and check the orientation of the articular surfaces to define the antetorsion (Fig. 9.9b).

A significant difference in penetration is the result of poor preparation, and if progression is too "easy", a diaphyseal fissure must be suspected

9.5.2 Implantation of the Definitive Proximal Part

- Carefully rinse the morse taper, it must always be perfectly clean. Position the proximal part by hand, and, before any impaction (even manual), regulate the antetorsion defined during the previous step (Fig. 9.10).
- Manual impaction and then definitive assembly with the torque wrench.

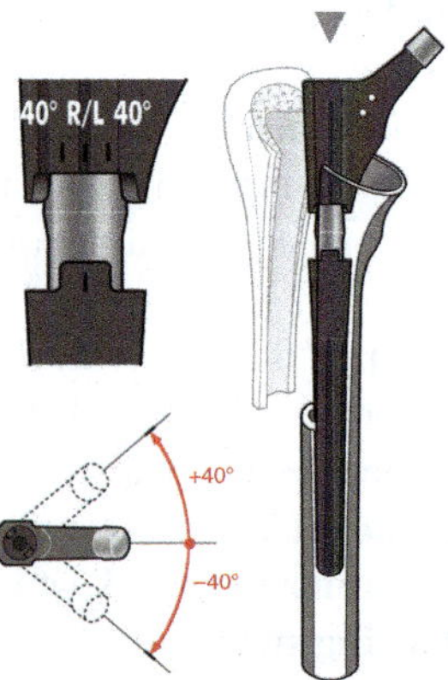

Fig. 9.10 Assembly of proximal part and adjust the antetorsion

To assemble the proximal and distal parts, follow the technique recommended for assembly, it is not advisable to use a hammer

When assembling the proximal part with the torque wrench, neutralize the torsional forces (see assembly technique)

- The safety nut is screwed into place, a trial femoral head (medium-sized neck) is placed and another reduction is performed.

NB: Before choosing the neck length for the definitive femoral head, check one last time if the progression of the implant is stopped by tapping on the shoulder of the prosthesis. If the implant subsides further (by 2 or 3 mm), this can be easily corrected if the trial reductions have been performed with a medium-sized trial neck.

9.6 Putting Flap Back into Place

Putting the flap back into place is an important and sometimes delicate moment of the surgery. It must be done carefully to prevent secondary gaps and to improve the primary stability of the implant.

- Eliminate all obstacles which are mostly situated at the level of the greater trochanter (corticalisation of the cancellous bone) and at the lower limit of the flap (endomedullary ossification) (Fig. 9.11).

If necessary, perform an osteotomy of the medial cortex to reduce the gaps at the level of the osteotomy lines and restore the contact with the implant.

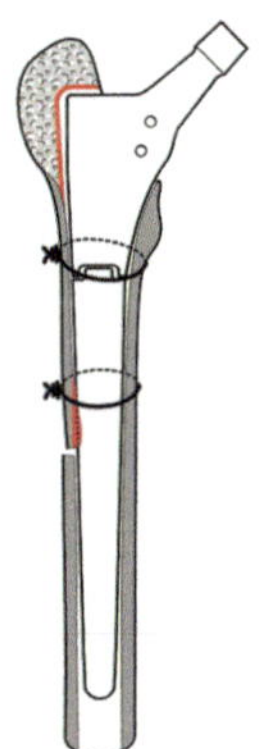

Fig. 9.11 Osteosynthesis of the flap with a double cerclage wire

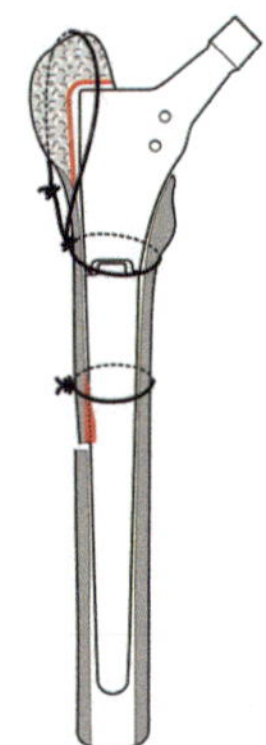

Fig. 9.12 Cerclage wire with lateral tension band

- Osteosynthesis of the flap is done with a double cerclage wire, or more, and by using the proximal cerclage to create an additional posterior and lateral tension band if the greater trochanter is weakened. This osteosynthesis is done with metal wires or cables (Fig. 9.12).

Reminder. It is possible to improve, or even ensure, the primary stability in the proximal region of the femur with a solid osteosynthesis on the flap if the cortices are of good quality and in contact with the implant. Avoid a cerclage that is too tight at the base of a weakened greater trochanter.

- Small bone defects can be neglected. If they are more extensive, in particular at the level of the osteotomy lines, it is possible to add autologous cortico-cancellous grafts.

Fractures of the flap usually have no negative consequences if the M. vastus lateralis remains fixed on the flap

9.7 Incidents

Faulty preparation of the anchorage zone after misjudging the femoral axis is often at the origin of incidents.

To avoid such incidents, it is important to observe the following rule: if you have the slightest doubt, make a new preparation of the femur and never make a forcible impaction

1. Crack or fracture in the diaphyseal region (Fig. 9.13) Such cracks or fractures are often at one of the two angles of the distal cut of the flap. When insertion of the implant is too easy or when no wedging is achieved at the planned level, you should suspect such an incident. In this case, remove the implant to apply one or two cerclage wires on the diaphyseal femur and make a new impaction, while constantly controlling that the gap at the level of the fracture is reduced. This minimal osteosynthesis is usually sufficient to ensure the stability of the prosthesis.

Such an incident can be avoided if the distal cut of the flap is delimited by two drill holes and if preventive (and most of the time definitive) cerclage wiring of the femur is performed when the cortices are weak

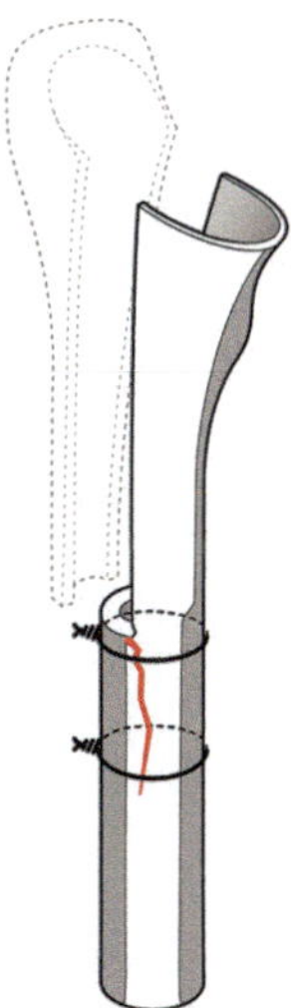

Fig. 9.13 Fracture: apply one or two cerclage wires

2. Prosthesis too high, reduction impossible or hip unstable

Such incidents are always the result of an "absent-minded" or too "hasty" surgeon who has not complied with the described operative protocol.

- *Prosthesis too high*. After assembly of the definitive proximal part, the prosthesis is too high and the reduction is difficult, or even impossible. In this case, disassemble the proximal component and select a less high proximal part. If this maneuver is impossible (55 mm high proximal part already in place), there is no other possibility than to remove the prosthesis from its seating to carry out an additional reaming or change the distal part. In this situation, the surgeon is often tempted by a forcible impaction, which merely results in jamming the prosthesis and making its removal even more difficult!
- *Reduction impossible* with a prosthesis implanted at the right level. Such an incident can occur if there is pronounced shortening of the lower limb with a very stiff hip in the beginning. After checking the degree of penetration of the inserted stem, perform an osteotomy of the linea aspera in the form of a decortication.

NB: In revision surgery, respecting strict equality of the length of the two lower limbs does not have to be an absolute dogma! It is necessary to avoid the impression of a too long leg often accepted with difficulty by the patient. This can be the case when there was significant shortening of the lower limb before revision.

- *Hip unstable*. It is advisable to intervene with regard to the height of the proximal component, and/or choose a retention cup and/or put the peri-articular muscles under tension by shortening the femoral flap.

3. Mobilization of the implant during the assembly of two prosthetic components

In such a case, remove the implant from its seat to correct its orientation and perform a new impaction while verifying the degree of penetration.

After this incident, if the prosthesis stabilizes in a lower position, and if it is not possible to correct this difference by a longer neck, it is necessary to change the height of the proximal part or ensure stabilization in the proximal region when putting the flap back into place and applying the cerclage wire on the flap.

Note: Several errors can be at the origin of this type of incident: deficient preparation of the anchorage zone, poor wedging of the prosthesis and/or the absence of a counter-pressure on the neck of the prosthesis during assembly of the two prosthetic parts with the torque wrench.

This option may be considered whenever the femur is straight in the frontal plane and when there are no significant bone defects.

Reminder: a femoral curvature in the frontal plane is always a contra-indication for an endofemoral approach, even if there are not bone defects.

- Ensure a perfect exteriorization of the femur because it is not possible to properly prepare a medullary cavity if the femur remains attached in the depth of the articular cavity.
- Wide opening of the greater trochanter to ensure that you are in the axis of the femoral diaphysis and to avoid implantation in varus position.
- Complete removal of the cement; this requires a perfect vision of the medullary canal and sometimes creating a femoral window.
- When preparing the femur and selecting the implant, make a good use of the modularity of the rasp/trial prosthesis. The objective is to ensure proximal fixation (mostly in the metaphyseo-diaphyseal zone) by means of a short stem.

10.1 Articular Approach(es)

The two articular approaches (antero-lateral and postero-lateral) can be used. However, the postero-lateral approach gives a more direct access to the main challenges associated with the implantation of a straight stem.

A small skin incision is possible; on the other hand, a mini-invasive articular approach with introduction of the implant via the femoral neck (or what remains of it!) is not recommended when a straight stem is chosen!

10.1.1 Postero-lateral Approach

The patient is placed in the lateral decubitus position. The pelvis is immobilized, dorsally by a sacral support, and ventrally by a public support (Fig. 10.1).

Avoid anterior compression of the femoral blood vessels

The lower limb is maintained horizontally by a cushion that can be easily moved so as not to hinder the hip adduction movements during luxation of the prosthesis and the exteriorization of the femur.

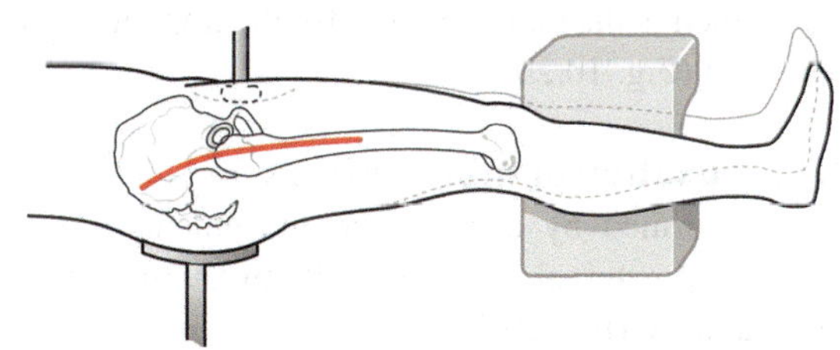

Fig. 10.1 Postero-lateral position and skin incision

10.1.1.1 Skin Incision

Skin incision centered on the greater trochanter, incision of the fascia lata and the gluteus maximus muscle in the direction of the muscular fibers.

Soft tissues are retracted with a distractor (Charnley type), which is both stable and rigid.

Avoid a skin incision too anterior or too posterior

P. Le Béguec et al., *Uncemented Femoral Stems for Revision Surgery*,
DOI 10.1007/978-3-319-03614-4_10, © Springer International Publishing Switzerland 2015

10.1.1.2 Articular Approach

- The posterior edge of the gluteus medius muscle is retracted after freeing its deep attachments at the tip of the greater trochanter.
- Posterior capsulotomy with section of the pyramidal and external rotator tendons close to the bone (Fig. 10.2a).

A section of the quadratus crural muscle and the aponevrotic extension of the gluteus maximus are often necessary

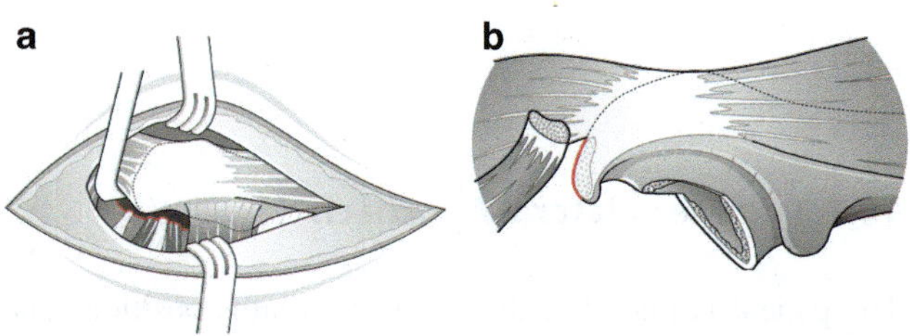

Fig. 10.2 Section of the pyramidal and external rotator tendons (**a**) and the posterior tendon of the gluteus medius muscle (**b**)

NB: A partial transverse section of the posterior tendon of the gluteus medius muscle (or detachment with a bone fragment) can prevent the muscular fibers from being lacerated during the preparation of the femur with a long reamer. It also ensures perfect exposition of the tip of the greater trochanter, which is the main obstacle for the implantation of a straight stem (Fig. 10.2b).

10.1.1.3 Luxation of the Prosthesis

This is performed by a combined movement of flexion, adduction and external rotation, while exerting traction on the femoral neck (Fig. 10.3).

When the hip is tight, proceed with caution, especially if the femur is weakened

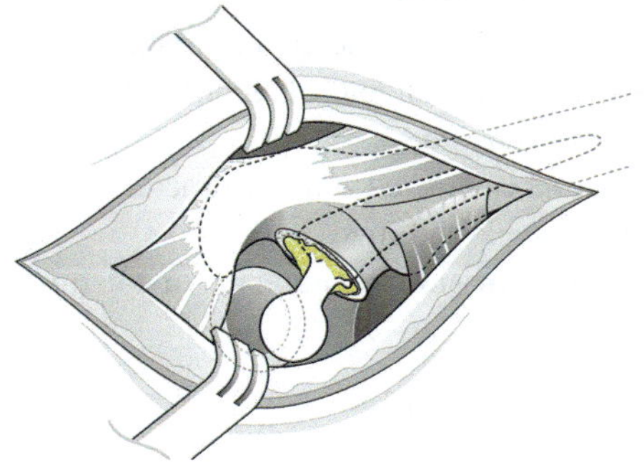

Fig. 10.3 Posterior luxation by flexion, adduction and external rotation

10.1.1.4 Removal of the Prosthesis

Make a lateral opening of the greater trochanter before removal of the femoral stem and ablation of the cement at the level of the shoulder of the stem (Fig. 10.4).

Removal of the prosthesis with an extractor that leans on the neck.

If prosthesis and cement form a block (loosening of bone and cement), make a wide opening of the greater trochanter

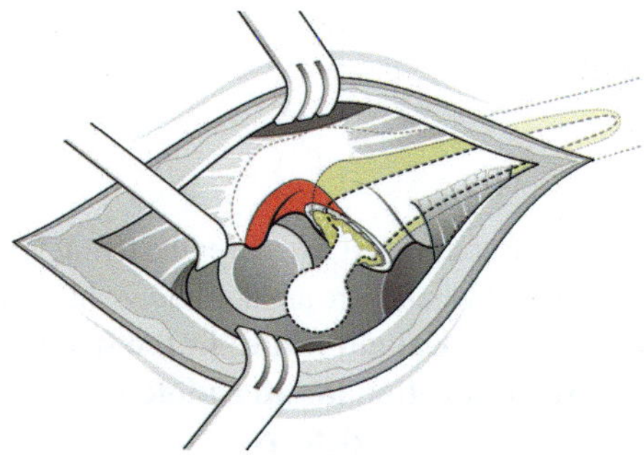

Fig. 10.4 Perform a wide opening of the greater trochanter

10.1.1.5 Exteriorization of the Femur

- Free the proximal femur from its fibrous and capsular attachments, particularly on the medial cortex and make sure to stay close to the bone.

The insertion point of a straight stem is situated at the level of the digital fossa (Fig. 10.5)

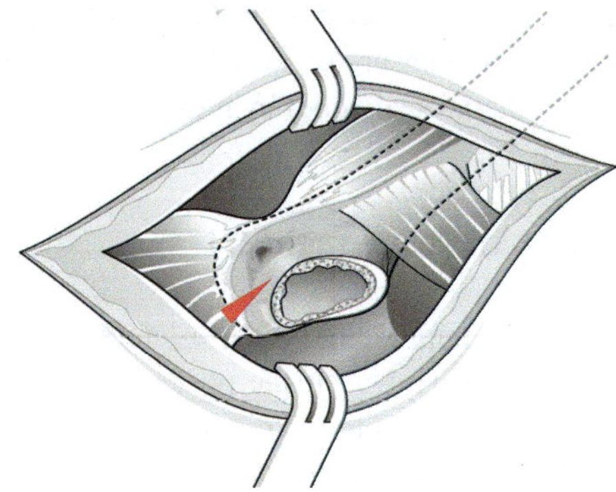

Fig. 10.5 Free the proximal femur to exteriorize the femur

- Excise fibrous tissues and granulomas in the articular cavity by proceeding from the center to the periphery to preserve the posterior capsule which protects the sciatic nerve.

Any attempt to exteriorize the femur by forcible adduction can lead to a fracture by avulsion of the proximal femur if it has not been detached beforehand

10.1.2 Antero-lateral Approach

The patient is placed in the dorsal decubitus position, with the hip to be operated protruding slightly over the edge of the table. The pelvis is stabilized by a wedge resting on the opposite hip.

10.1.2.1 Skin Incision
- Lateral skin incision centered on the greater trochanter, slightly angled upward and forward at the level of the pelvis (Fig. 10.6).
  Avoid a too anterior skin incision
- Incision of the facia lata and the gluteus maximus muscle in the direction of the muscular fibers. Soft tissues are retracted with a rigid distractor (Charnley type).

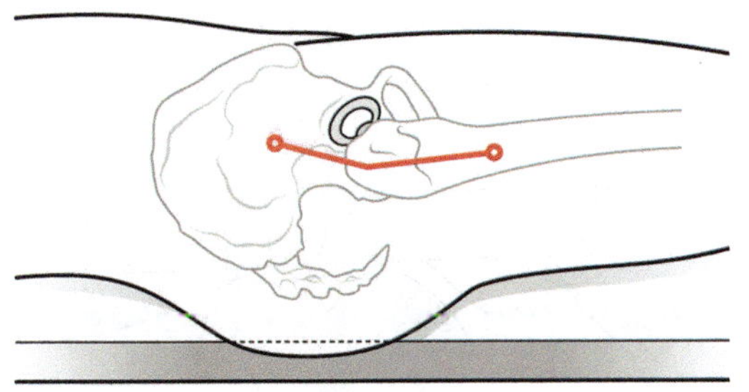

Fig. 10.6 Antero-lateral approach: skin incision

10.1.2.2 Articular Approach
- Incision of the transgluteal and digastric muscle with the vastus lateralis. Section of the tendon and muscle, staying close to the bone and at distance from the superior gluteal nerve (Fig. 10.7).
  Avoid a too anterior detachment of the digastric muscle to preserve its anatomic continuity
- All these tissues are retracted with an auto-static distractor (Charnley type) that was previously set up.
- Perform an anterior capsulotomy or capsulectomy if the hip is tight.

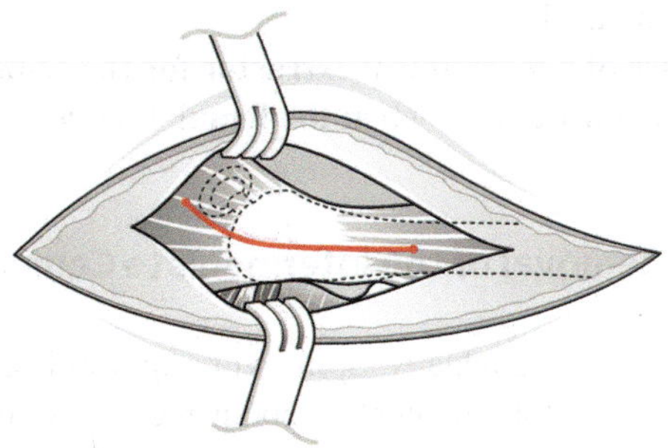

Fig. 10.7 Transgluteal and digastric muscle with the vastus lateralis

10.1.2.3 Luxation of the Prosthesis
This is performed by a combined movement of flexion, adduction and external rotation, while exerting traction on the femoral neck (Fig. 10.8).

Before any attempt of luxation, if the hip is tight, free the articular cavity to obtain decoaptation of the articular surfaces by traction on the lower limb

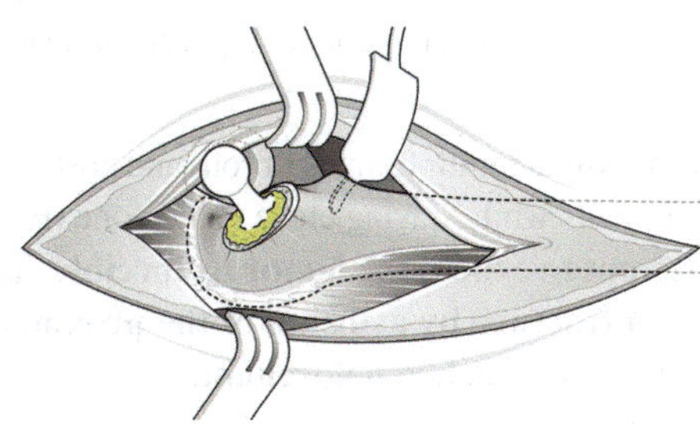

Fig. 10.8 Antero-lateral luxation by flexion, adduction and external rotation

10.1.2.4 Removal of the Prosthesis
Make a lateral opening of the greater trochanter before removal of the femoral stem and ablation of the cement at the shoulder of the stem (Fig. 10.9).

Removal of the prosthesis with an extractor that leans on the neck.

If prosthesis and cement form a block (loosening between bone and cement), make a wide opening of the greater trochanter

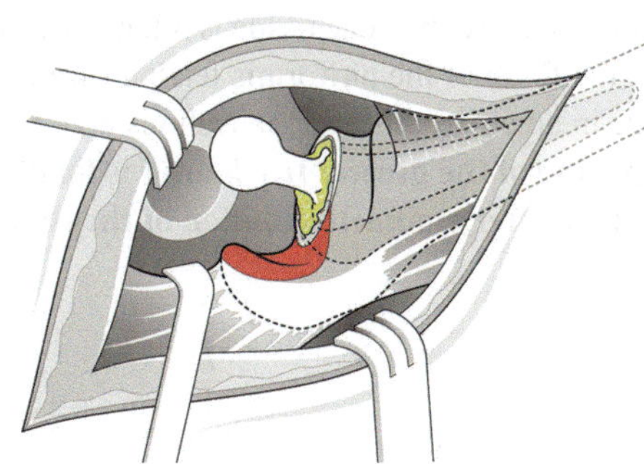

Fig. 10.9 Lateral opening of the greater trochanter before removal prosthesis

10.1.2.5 Exteriorization of the Femur
If an anterolateral approach has been chosen, the exteriorization of the femur is a particularly important moment of the surgery, particularly when the hip is tight.
- Excise fibrous tissues and granulomas from the articular cavity.

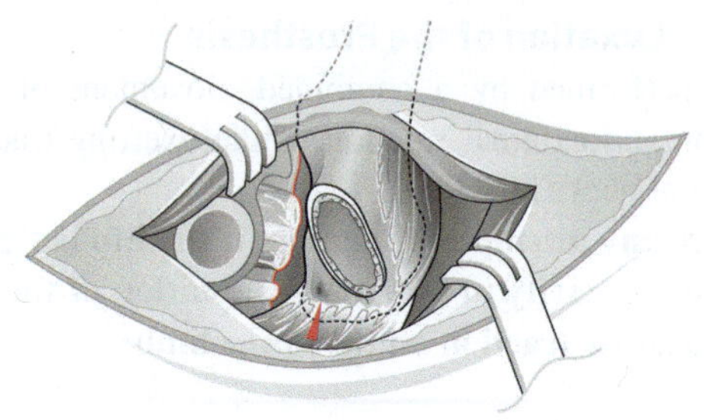

Fig. 10.10 Free the fibrous and posterior capsular attachments

- Free the proximal femur from its fibrous and posterior capsular attachments while staying close to the bone (Fig. 10.10).

Any attempt to expose the femur by forcible adduction can lead to a fracture by avulsion of the proximal femur if it has not been detached beforehand

10.2　Femoral Approach(es)

10.2.1　Opening of the Greater Trochanter

- An endofemoral approach implies a wide opening of the greater trochanter (Fig. 10.11) as a straight revision stem (which is also sometimes long) must follow the path of a centro-medullary nail.

The penetration point of a straight stem is situated at the level of the digital fossa

- After ablation of the proximal cement and before continuing the removal in the intermediate and distal zones of the femur, make a lateral and posterior opening of the greater trochanter because the bone tissue is often dense and sclerotic at the fossa of the piriformis tendon (use bone chisels to be in an environment of cancellous bone).

The opening of the greater trochanter is finalized with a long reamer after complete ablation of the cement

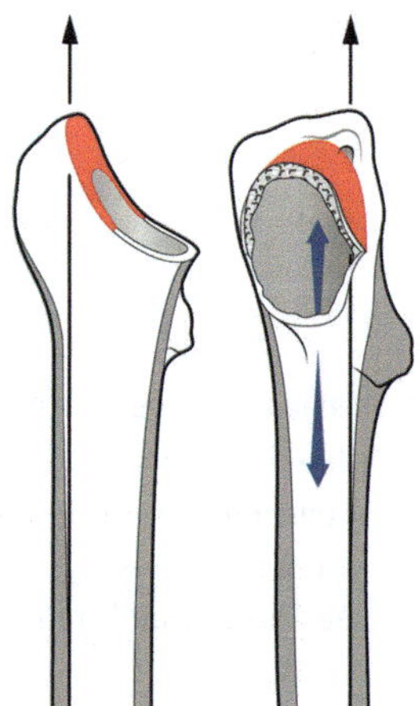

Fig. 10.11 Great trochanter: opening lateral and posterior

10.2.2　Trochanteric Osteotomy

A trochanteric osteotomy performed before or after ablation of the implant constitutes, at the same time, an articular and a femoral approach (Fig. 10.12).

- A trochanteric osteotomy is proposed when the hip is tight, in the presence of a curvature of the proximal femur (after an inter-trochanteric osteotomy) and if, moreover, proximal fixation is strongly desirable.
- This is a digastric trochanteric osteotomy with preservation of the insertions of the vastus lateralis muscle which have an important role for the secondary stability of the greater trochanter.

The indications for a trochanteric osteotomy are not frequent. We often recommend a femorotomy in the form of a flap

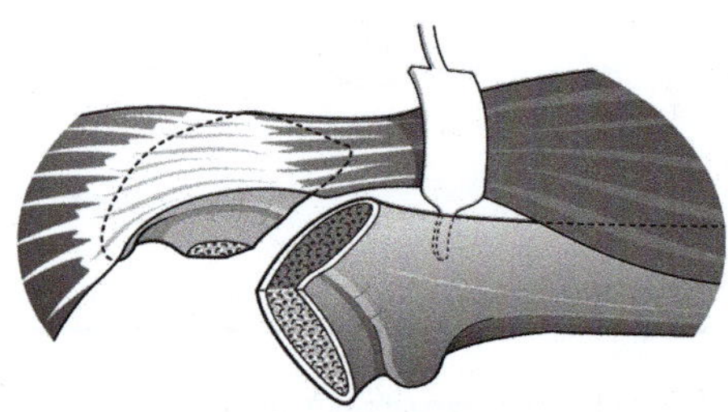

Fig. 10.12 Digastric trochanteric osteotomy

10.3　Cement Removal

The removal of the cement must always be complete when an uncemented stem has been chose. This is often tedious work if the cortices are weakened and, thus, for many surgeons a good reason to perform a femoral flap.

A perfect vision of the endomedullary space is indispensible: (1) wide opening of the greater trochanter, (2) take into account a femoral curvature (sagittal plane), even if is not very accentuated.

The use of a mechanical extractor for the cement does not prevent a via falsa when the femur is curved!

10.3.1　Removal of the Intermediate Cement

The cement is gradually split with appropriate chisels (Fig. 10.13). At any moment a good perception of the bone/cement interface is indispensable, which requires a careful curettage of the granulomas and fibrous tissue.

Cold light and extensive rinsing with aspiration are necessary at this point of the surgery

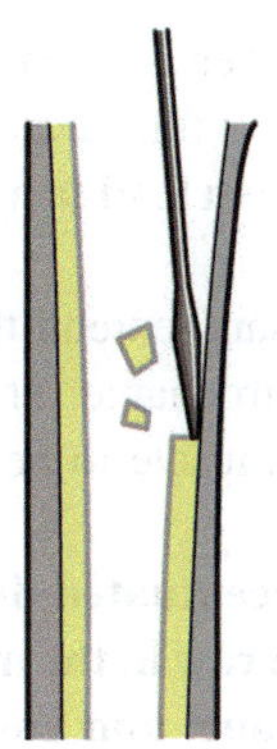

Fig. 10.13 Removal of intermediate cement

10.3.2 Removal of the Distal Cement Plug

Following the removal of the intermediate cement, the distal cement is ablated.

- With a 6 mm diameter drill, drill a hole in the cement plug, making sure that it is properly centered (Fig. 10.14a).
- Ensure that there is no via falsa, then gradually increase the diameter of the drill to 10 or 11 mm to be able to use a wide extractor that serves as a rake. This instrument is particularly efficient to remove the remaining cement (Fig. 10.14b).

Take into account an eccentric position of the distal tip of the stem

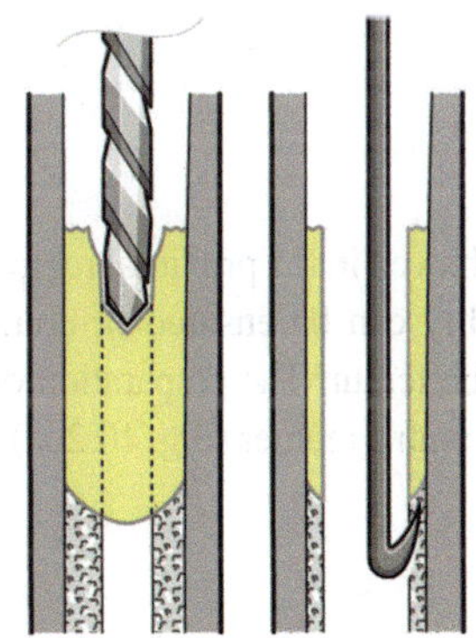

Fig. 10.14 Pierce the plug and excision of the cement with an extractor

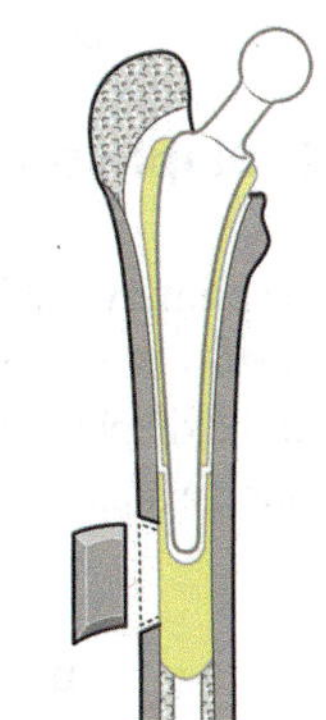

Fig. 10.15 Femoral window

A femoral window may be recommended to remove a cement plug while preserving the possibility of proximal fixation of the implant.

Depending on the articular approach that is chosen, the window can be lateral or antero-lateral. If the cortices are thick, it can be performed in the shape of a "wedge", which makes it easier to put it back into place – most of the time without osteosynthesis (Fig. 10.15).

Avoid a perpendicular position of the chisels on the cortices during the ablation of the distal cement

10.4 Calibrating the Femur

- After complete ablation of the cement, calibrate the medullary canal with a cylindrical reamer to eliminate a narrowing zone at the tip of prosthesis (Fig. 10.16a).

A residual cement fragment or an endomedullary ossification can result in eccentric reaming or even a via falsa (Fig. 10.16b)

- Use a tapered and long reamer of a diameter smaller than that of the medullary canal to check the alignment of the proximal femur in comparison with the diaphyseal femur. Adjust the opening of the greater trochanter in its lateral and posterior zones (Fig. 10.16c).

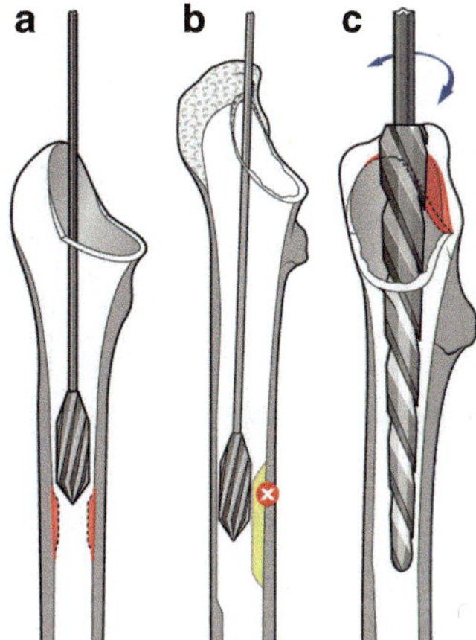

Fig. 10.16 Calibrate the medullary canal (**a**) avoid an eccentric reaming (**b**) adjust the opening of the greater trochanter (**c**)

10.5 Preparation of the Anchorage Zone

- In principle, seek proximal fixation (often metaphyseo-diaphyseal). The preparation of the femur is done with the rasps that also serve as trial prostheses.
- If a proximal fixation is impossible or precarious, seek a short additional fixation in the diaphyseal region. In this case, the use of reamers is necessary and the rasp only serves as trial prosthesis.

10.5.1 Proximal Fixation (in the Metaphyseo-Diaphyseal Zone)

A *modular rasp*, which is also a trial prosthesis, makes a preparation of the femur in two stages possible.

1. Assemble the distal rasp, length 120 mm, Ø14 mm (if narrow femur +) or length 140 mm, Ø14, 16 or 18 mm (if wider femur), with a cylindrical and graduated handle.
   - The distal rasp is impacted until primary stability is obtained (Fig. 10.17).
   - Evaluate the degree of penetration. The tip of the greater trochanter serves as a reference.

Example: a reference **1–65** corresponds to a distal rasp of length 120 or 140 mm (number **1**), coupled with a proximal rasp of height **65** mm. Avoid using a proximal component of 55 or 85 mm (or 105 if complete range) to keep some flexibility when choosing the definitive implant.

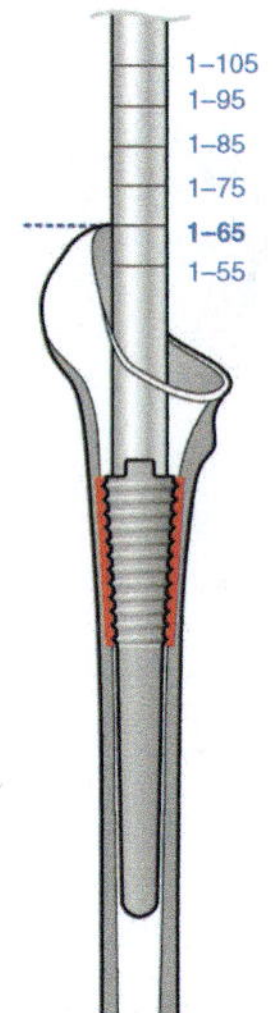

Fig. 10.17 Distal rasp for the metaphyseo-diaphyseal zone

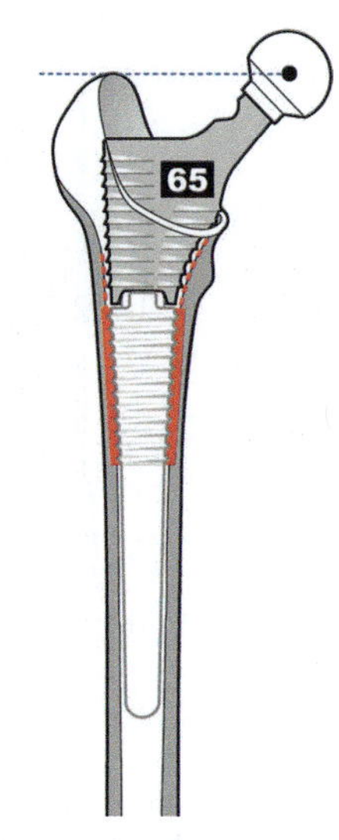

Fig. 10.18 Trial prosthesis with distal and proximal rasp

If the primary stability is not perfect, make a new attempt after assembly of the proximal part (see here after) before opting for additional diaphyseal fixation

2. Assemble the distal rasp and the proximal rasp whose height has been determined during the previous surgical step. The assembly is impacted into the medullary canal by light hammer blows.

   Check the degree of penetration of the rasp/test prosthesis: the center of rotation and the tip of the greater trochanter must be aligned (Fig. 10.18).

   NB. If difficulties occur at this point of the surgery, it is possible to make a separate preparation of the metaphysis with a smaller proximal rasp, if needed, and without using a distal part.

   For the Revitan® system, choose a tulip-shaped proximal component and a distal component of length 120 or 140 mm (diameters 14 and 16 mm are most frequently used)

3. The greater trochanter is often the cause of difficulties during insertion, and, in fine, a varus position (Fig. 10.19).

Forcible impaction can lead to a fracture of the greater trochanter

Verify and, if necessary, extend the lateral and posterior opening of the greater trochanter at the level of the digital fossa of the piriformis muscle to be insured to work in the axis of the femur.

A femur with an accentuated double curvature in the sagittal view can be narrow in the metaphyseo-diaphyseal zone of the sagittal plane, and complementary reaming can be necessary

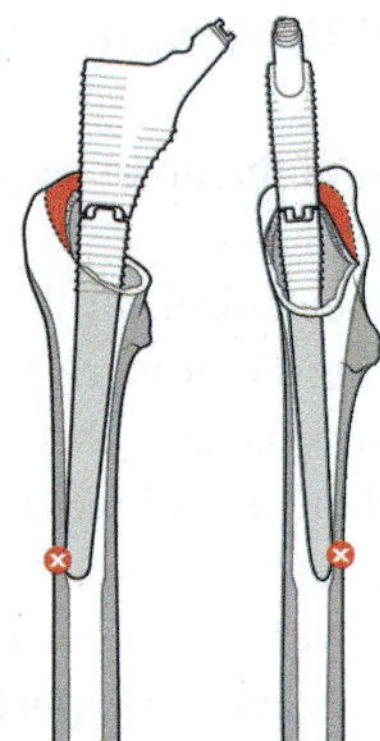

Fig. 10.19 Wide opening lateral and posterior of the greater trochanter

10.5.2 Diaphyseal Fixation

When the primary stability is not achieved in the proximal region or if it seems precarious, the stability can be ensured or completed in the diaphyseal region of the femur. The preparation of the anchorage area is then achieved with a reamer (Fig. 10.20a).

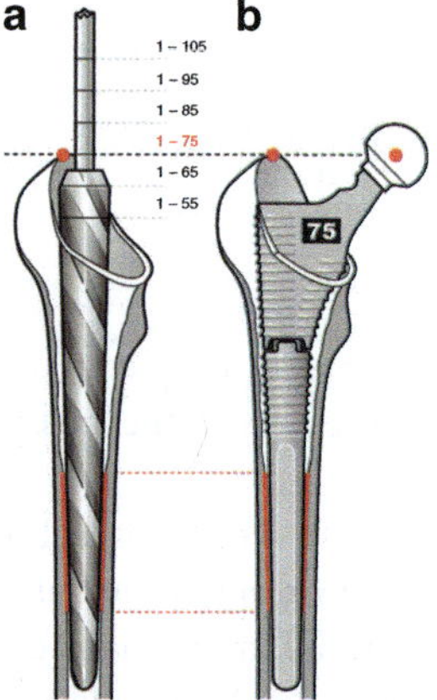

Fig. 10.20 Reaming of the femur (**a**) and choosing of the implant with a trial prosthesis (**b**)

- Gradually increase the diameter of the reamer until you obtain good stability (the reamer does not advance any further).
- Check on the inserted handle of the reamer the mark that is aligned with, or in the immediate vicinity, of the tip of the greater trochanter. The reamer must be in zone 1 (distal part of length 140 mm) and accommodate a proximal part of medium height (avoid the extreme heights 55 or 85 mm or 105 mm, if complete range)

If the reamer is in zone 2 (distal part of length 200 mm) increase the diameter of the reamer

Example: a reference of **1–75** corresponds to a trial prosthesis of the same diameter as the inserted reamer and a distal part of length 140 mm (number **1**), coupled with a proximal part of height **75** mm (Fig. 10.20b).

10.6 Selection of the Definitive Implant

Assembly of the two components of the trial prosthesis determined during the previous surgical step (length/diameter of the distal part and height of the proximal part) and selection of a femoral head with a medium neck.

In the case of an endofemoral approach, it is not possible to proceed to an implantation in two stages, and the only safety margin left to the surgeon when implanting the definitive stem is the length of the neck

The assembled component is inserted in the medullary canal and impacted by light hammer blows while checking the antetorsion. Verify the degree of penetration by taking the tip of the greater trochanter as reference. Three situations can occur:

10.6.1 Reduction Is Easy

The articular surfaces are stable and oriented correctly, and the length of the lower limb is restored: the chosen prosthesis is the right one (note the degree of antetorsion of the definitive proximal component).

If the definitive stem subsides slightly more, or less deeply, than the trial prosthesis, this difference can be corrected when selecting the definitive femoral head.

10.6.2 Reduction Is Difficult or Even Impossible

This situation can occur if the lower limb was far shorter and/or the hip very stiff prior to surgery. In such cases, perfect compensation of leg length discrepancy is sometimes difficult to achieve, and it is often preferable to make an under-correction to avoid the impression of a lower limb that is too long, which is generally poorly tolerated by the patient.

- If the choice of a short neck is not sufficient, it is necessary to decrease the height of the proximal part. If this is also not an option, it is necessary to ream further.
- The prosthesis is implanted at a correct level and it is not possible to consider a lower implantation. In this case, if the reduction is difficult or even impossible, perform an osteotomy of the linea aspera, in combination with the classic steps of an intra-articular release.

10.6.3 Reduction Is Too Easy and the Hip Is Unstable

This is often due to a severe muscular deficiency. In these cases, it is often preferable and more efficient to opt for a retention cup or a cup with dual mobility to avoid the risk of a lower limb that is too long or a recurrent dislocation!

10.7 Implantation of the Definitive Stem

1. Assembly of the two prosthetic components with a torque wrench outside the femur by adjusting the desired antetorsion for the proximal component

   It is not recommended to assemble the components in situ when using an endofemoral approach because the risks of poor assembly are too high
2. Manually introduce the prosthesis into the medullary cavity by giving it the appropriate orientation (avoid correction of the antetorsion during the impaction).

   If the prosthesis is too exterior, this is often due to insufficient preparation of the anchorage area

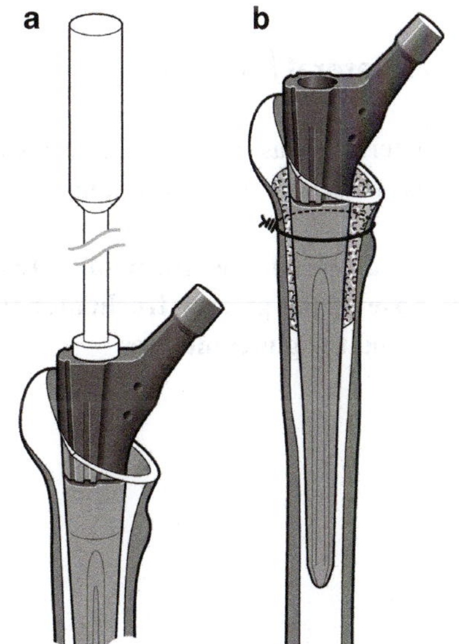

Fig. 10.21 With a impactor wedge the prosthesis (**a**) and if necessary inserting cortico-spongious grafts (**b**)

With the help of an impactor screwed into the proximal part (Fig. 10.21a), wedge the prosthesis by light hammer blows, over a distance of about 2–4 cm, until a cortical sound is obtained. Diligently check the progression of the implant. Assess stability, wait a few minutes and check again whether the implant has settled and progression has stopped.

Avoid forcible impaction (risk of fracture). If the progression of the implant is too "easy", make sure that there is no cortical fracture

NB. By inserting intra-medullary cortico-spongious grafts, it is possible to control or even limit the penetration of the prosthesis, and at the same time improve its stability. Bone grafting must be done before final impaction of the prosthesis or after taking the implant a couple of centimeters out of its seating (Fig. 10.21b).

3. Selection of a trial femoral head (medium size), reduction and control of the length of the two lower limbs and the stability of the hip.
4. Selection of the appropriate length of the definitive femoral head

10.8 Articular Closure

10.8.1 Posterolateral Approach

The pelvitrochanteric muscle and the posterior capsule are reattached to the posterior edge of the greater trochanter and the posterior fibers of the gluteus medius muscle once the latter has been attached to the tip of the great trochanter by two or three trans-osseous points, if it has been sectioned.

10.8.2 Anterolateral Approach

Reattach the anterior digastric muscle (gluteus medius and vastus lateralis muscles) with two trans-osseous points (Fig. 10.22).

Additional fixation in the form of a tension band between the base of the greater trochanter (by a transosseous point) and the glutei muscles

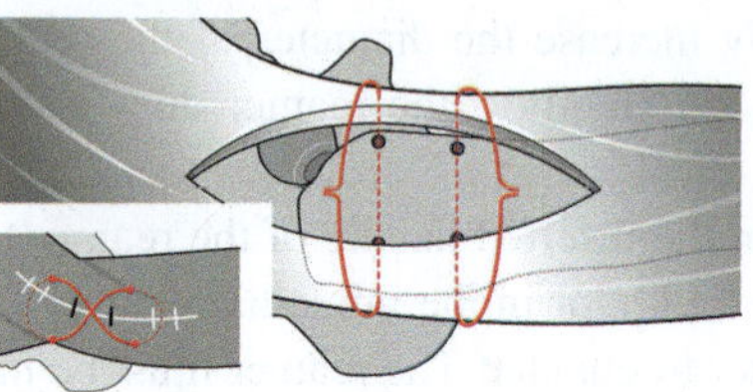

Fig. 10.22 Closure of the anterolateral approach with two transosseous points

10.8.3 Greater Trochanter

Before reattaching the great trochanter, ensure that there is no cement left at this level. If necessary, remodel the endomedullary side of the greater trochanter to obtain a perfect application on the shoulder of the prosthesis.

- If a digastric osteotomy has been performed, apply a lateral and posterior cerclage wire, in the form of a tension band, between the proximal femur and the glutei muscles. This can be enough to neutralize the tensile stresses exerted by the glutei muscles and the vastus lateralis upward and forward (Fig. 10.23).

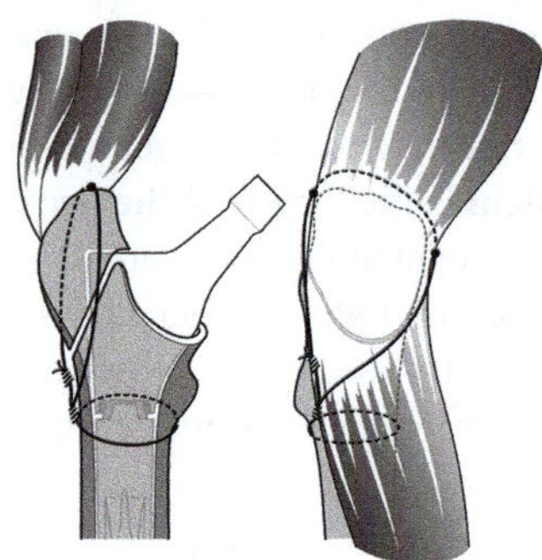

Fig. 10.23 If digastric osteotomy: apply a lateral and posterior cerclage wire

- For a classic trochanteric osteotomy with desinsertion of the vastus lateralis, perform an osteosynthesis with three metal wires and complete it by a metal wire that form a lateral tension band

A fracture of the greater trochanter is treated in the same way

Main Objectives

Generally speaking, one should not be overly cautious or ambiguous, and at first, physiotherapy should be exclusively functional.

- **Being overly cautious** means keeping the patient in bed in traction and suspension for several weeks. If the technique adopted by the surgeon generally requires such measures, not only the reliability of the method must be questioned, but also its consequences, both economically and for the patient!

- **An ambiguous attitude** consists in giving the patient permission to return home with instructions of complete unloading, or – even more dangerous – of partial weight-bearing. Once the post-operative pain has waned, the patient will probably be tempted to test the solidity of the prosthesis, which, in the absence of pain, often results in complete loading too soon after surgery.

Concerning Rehabilitation

Immediate postoperative instructions for the patient should be simple and pragmatic. We can distinguish two different situations:

1. The prosthesis is stable

The prosthesis is stable and has perfectly wedged in a femur with thick cortices and in a tapered medullary canal.

In this situation, immediate loading with the help of two crutches is permitted. The crutches play a double role: they relieve the hip and avoid faulty moves until the soft tissues have completely healed. Immediate postoperative physiotherapy is only functional and aims at teaching the patient which moves to avoid in order to protect the prosthesis from rotational stresses. This is particularly important when standing up from a seated position or when walking up or down stairs.

The patient consults again 2 months after surgery, at which point also a follow-up radiograph is done. At that moment, a more active physiotherapy can be prescribed, if necessary. Depending on the recovery of the muscular strength and knowing that crutches must not be dropped too quickly, all support is gradually dropped.

2. The prosthesis is not stable

The surgeon has a doubt with regard to the primary stability of the implant.

Whatever the reasons for this concern, it is advisable to exercise caution and not to authorize weight-bearing, even partial, during a period of 6 weeks.

Every patient is unique. Often, the period of non-loading can be reduced to approximately 4 weeks

During the period of non-loading, it is better to keep the patient under surveillance and, if he is placed in a specialized rehabilitation center, no active physiotherapy should be done during this time. At the end of this period and after a follow-up radiograph, weight-bearing is permitted; it should really be progressive, but in reality, patients generally take up full weight-bearing immediately.

This careful approach is recommended in the beginning of the learning curve and until the surgeon masters the surgical technique

Part IV

Evaluation of Radiographic Results – How?

The method described below is based on **three principles**:

1. **Propose a universal method**, i.e. usable for all uncemented revision stems and for primary surgery, independent of their concept.

2. **Make a numerical evaluation** to better rank the various chosen criteria and facilitate a comparative study. The advantages of this approach are that it limits the risks of an evaluation that is too subjective and makes a comparative study more reliable.

3. **Perform two separate evaluations**:
   (a) Evaluation of initial and secondary bone stock.
   (b) Evaluation of osseointegration and secondary stability.

The **G**lobal **R**adiological **S**core is a synthesis of the evaluation of secondary bone stock and secondary stability.

Warning!
This fourth part only applies to the radiographic results obtained by the proposed method. This study does not include all means to evaluate a result, there is especially no reference to survival curves and other indices of patient satisfaction.

This evaluation concerns the initial (or immediately postoperative) bone stock and the secondary bone stock. It takes into account all bone modifications arising in the contact with an uncemented implant and, more particularly, the regeneration of the cortices in revision cases. These two successive evaluations are performed by using the same criteria.

11.1 Method

- On an immediate postoperative a/p radiograph, Gruen zones 1, 2, 3, 5 and 6 [24] are successively and separately evaluated, knowing that zone 7, often absent in revision, is integrated to zone 6. The bone density, the thickness of the cortices and the presence of a bone defect are assessed. This first evaluation is used as a reference to estimate the secondary bone stock and to study the factors that could have an impact on the final result (secondary bone stock and secondary stability).

- At the last follow-up, on a second postoperative a/p radiograph, we do the same evaluation to determine whether the bone stock around the femoral implant is preserved, regenerated, or, to the contrary, whether it has degraded. Only the evaluation of the secondary bone stock is taken into account to establish the **G**lobal **R**adiological **S**core.

Table 11.1 Post operative bone stock: 1-immediate 2-secondary

Evaluation zone 1 (G.T.)		Evaluation zone 7
O 4 No damage		Evaluation integrated into zone 6
O 2 Moderate damage		
O 0 Severe damage		
O –2 Cortical lysis		
Evaluation zone 2		**Evaluation zone 6**
O 4 No damage		No damage 4 O
O 2 Moderate damage		Moderate damage 2 O
O 0 Severe damage		Severe damage 0 O
O –2 Cortical lysis		Cortical lysis –2 O
Evaluation zones 3		**Evaluation zone 5**
O 4 No damage		No damage 4 O
O 2 Moderate damage		Moderate damage 2 O
O 0 Severe damage		Severe damage 0 O
O –2 Cortical lysis		Cortical lysis –2 O

Total-1 /20 O Very good (20–18); O Good (16–14); O Average (12–10); O Poor (<10)
Total-2 /20 O Very good (20–18); O Good (16–14); O Average (12–10); O Poor (<10)

P. Le Béguec et al., *Uncemented Femoral Stems for Revision Surgery*,
DOI 10.1007/978-3-319-03614-4_11, © Springer International Publishing Switzerland 2015

11.1.1 Cortical Modifications

11.1.1.1 Thickness of the Cortices

On a preoperative a/p radiograph, the thickness of the cortices in a non-implanted femoral zone (isthmic zone) is taken as a reference. If the revision concerns a long stem, this is done on the contra-lateral femur. In zone 1 (greater trochanter), the thickness concerns the cortices and the underlying spongy tissue.

- Any significant decrease of the cortical thickness without modification of the bone density is taken into account immediately after surgery or at the last follow-up.

  Decrease of the cortical thickness associated with a decrease of bone density is evaluated at the level of the bone density to avoid assessing the same parameter twice.

- In the context of a revision, they are often the consequence of granulomas, abnormal mobility of the implant, or, more rarely, of iatrogenic origin (eccentric reaming).
- More rarely, at the last follow-up, cortical modifications take the form of cortical thickening which can be associated with an increase of the bone density (only the cortical thickening is taken into account). Such modifications are due to an anomaly in load transmission and they are less pejorative than a decrease of the bone density or cortical thickness when a new intervention become necessary.

11.1.1.2 Bone Density

This evaluation concerns all decreases of bone density in the context of an uncemented implant which can be attributed to non-solicitation of the femoral cortices (absence of tensile and compressive stresses). This evaluation is based on the presence or absence of a trabecular aspect of the cortical bone [21] and a comparison of the grey levels on two consecutive radiographs, according to the method described in Appendix 2. A classification is established depending on the decrease of bone density (moderate or severe), its extent and the presence or not of a decrease of cortical thickness.

11.1.1.3 Defects of the Cortical Bone

This evaluation concerns specifically revisions. Only the loss of bone substance in the form of an inter-fragmentary gap, following a fracture or a trochantero-diaphyseal femorotomy (distal cut of a flap or a femoral window), or an osteotomy of the medial cortex are taken into account.

Note: The loss of cortical bone substance, which is often a consequence of granulomas or a secondary necrosis, is taken into account in the evaluation of the cortices.

When 2 types of different lesions affect the same zone (inter-fragmentary gap and decrease cortical thickness), only the more unfavourable value is taken into account.

11.1.2 Evaluation of Cortical Lesions

A numerical score, from +4 to −2 points, is given for every Gruen zone. The final score is based on 20 points and the classification made in four categories: very good (20–18); good (16–14); average (12–10); poor (<10).

For each qualitative stage, a numerical mean is calculated.

Table 11.2 Evaluation of cortical lesions

+4	Any initial lesion or complete regeneration (density and thickness)
+2	Moderated decrease density or thickness or défect ≤ in 10 mm[a]
0	Severe decrease density or thickness or défect >10 mm[b]
−2	Major decrease density and thickness or cortical lysis (lysis of the G.T)

[a]Or increase thickness
[b]Or pseudarthrosis of the greater trochanter

+4 Pts   no initial lesions, nor secondary degradation, or complete regeneration of the cortices and/or filling of bone defects. No decrease of the bone density.

+2 Pts   moderate decrease of the cortical thickness, initially considered normal or incomplete regeneration of a severe initial lesion of the cortices, or bone defect <10 mm (secondary appearance or initial defect not filled), or moderate decrease of the bone density (normal thickness of cortices), or increased thickness of the cortices in zones 3 and/or 5 (special case).

0 Pts   severe decrease of the cortical thickness or no regeneration of an initial damage rated as severe and no decrease of the bone density, or marked decrease of the bone density and cortical thickness not modified or bone defect =/>10 mm (secondary appearance or initial defect not filled), or pseudarthrosis of the greater trochanter after osteotomy or fracture.

−2 Pts   major lesions: strong decrease of the density and thickness of the cortices or lysis of cortices or of the greater trochanter or initial bone defect aggravated.

11.2 Results (Figs. 11.1, 11.2, 11.3, 11.4, 11.5, and 11.6)

11.2.1 Global Results

- For the results rated as very good-good and the cases evaluated as average-poor, the differences between initial and secondary bone stock are not significant: 70% versus 67% for very good-good cases and 30% versus 33% for average-poor cases (p=0.5). The benefits achieved by a significant increase of the cases with secondary bone stock rated as very good (44% versus 25%) were largely offset by a net increase of cases rated as poor (15% versus 5%).

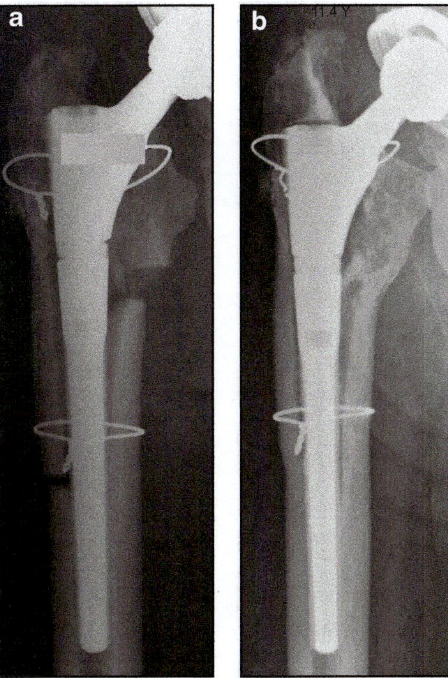

Fig. 11.1 A 69-year-old male patient. Revision by means of a transfemoral approach and osteotomy of the medial cortex. Initial bone stock evaluated at 14/20 (lesion of the greater trochanter ± and bone gaps) (a). Results at 11 years: filling of bone defects, secondary bone stock evaluated as very good: 18/20 (b)

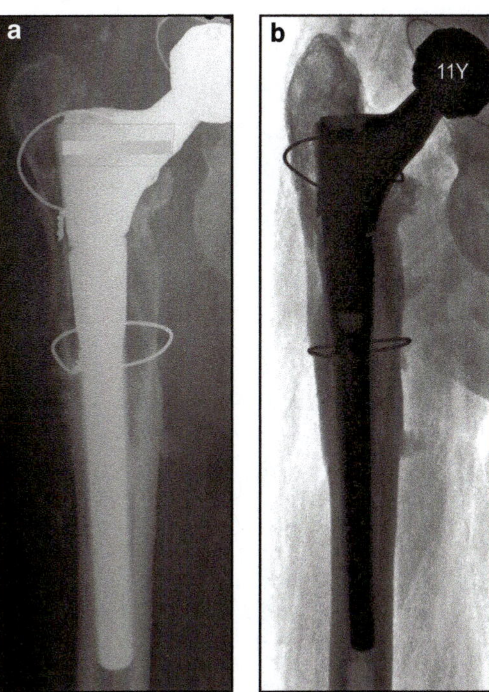

Fig. 11.2 A 52-year-old male patient. Revision by means of a transfemoral approach, lesions in zones 1, 2 and 6, initial bone stock evaluated at 12/20 (a). Results at 11 years: very good bone regeneration, secondary bone stock rated as very good: 18/20 (persistence of a discreet bone defect in zone 2) (b)

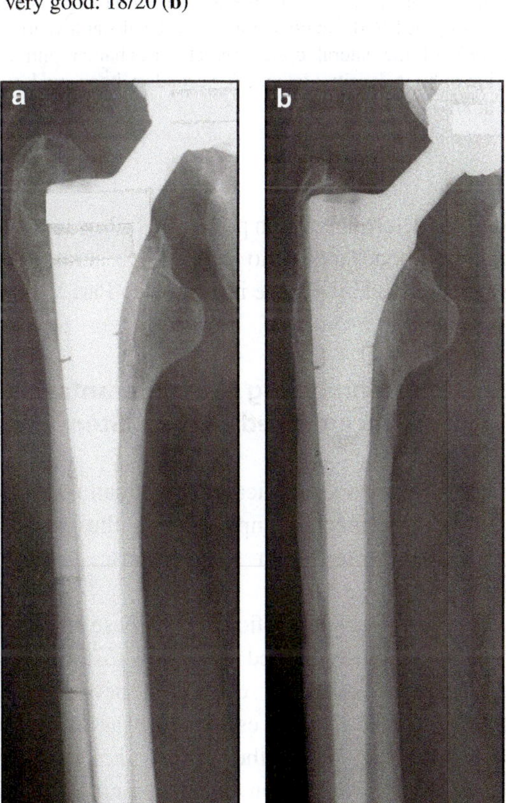

Fig. 11.3 A 70-year-old male patient. Revision by endofemoral approach and femoral window. Initial bone stock evaluated as very good at 18/20 (a). Results at 8 years: degradation ++ of the greater trochanter and secondary bone stock evaluated as good + at 16/20 (b)

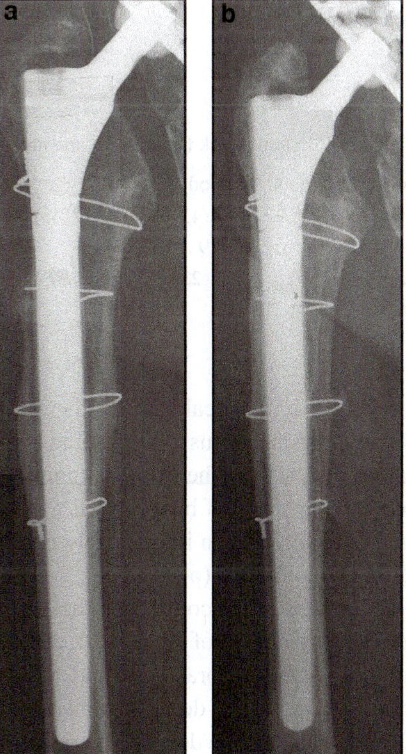

Fig. 11.4 A 61-year-old female patient. Revision by transfemoral approach. Lesions of lateral cortex +. Initial bone stock evaluated as average at 10/20, no bone grafts (a). Results at 5 years: regeneration of the lateral cortex except in zone 3, medial cortex stable, secondary bone stock evaluated as good – at 14/20 (b). **NB**. No secondary subsidence, lateral pedestal

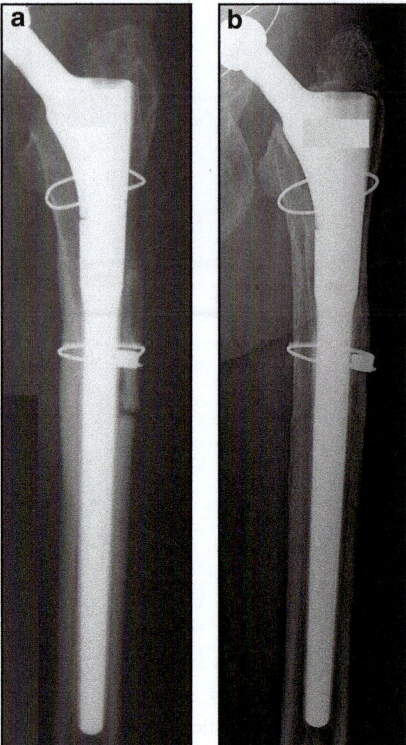
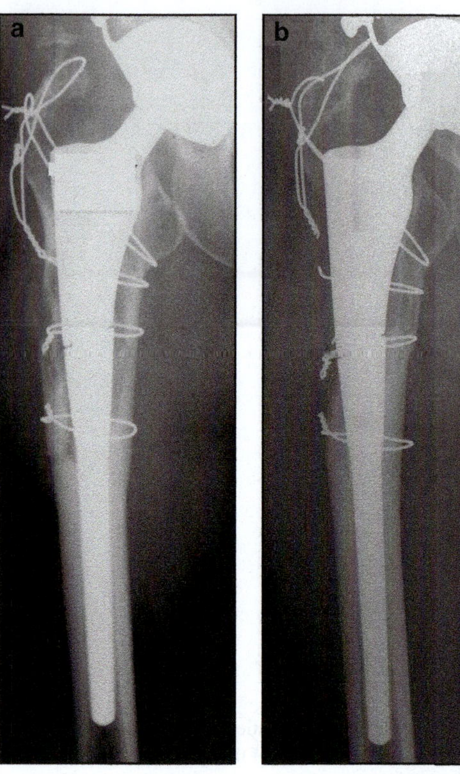

Fig. 11.5 A 71-year-old female patient. Revision by transfemoral approach. Lesions in zones 2+, 6± and 3±. Initial bone stock evaluated as good at 14/20. No bone grafts (**a**). Results at 7 years: degradation+ of the greater trochanter. No regeneration in zone 2 and diminution of thickness and density of the cortex in zone 3. Secondary bone stock evaluated as average at 10/20 (**b**)

Fig. 11.6 A 69-year-old female patient. Revision by transfemoral approach. Lesions in zones 1 and 2++ and 6±. Initial bone stock evaluated as average at 12/20. No bone grafts (**a**). Results at 8 years: secondary necrosis of the lateral cortex (greater trochanter and zone 2), diminution of bone density± in zone 6. Secondary bone stock evaluated as poor at 8/20 (**b**)

Table 11.3 Evaluation bone stock (*qualitative and numerical value*)

Bone stock	Very good	Good	Average	Poor
Initial bone stock	38 (25%)	67 (45%)	38 (25%)	7 (5%)
	18.5	14.9	11.1	7
Secondary bone stock	**66 (44%)**	**34 (23%)**	**27 (18%)**	**23 (15%)**
	18.3	**15**	**11.4**	**5.5**

- Translation into a numerical value of the results obtained in qualitative version seems coherent and confirms a first observation: in the end, there is no significant improvement of the mean value of bone capital which is globally estimated to be 14, 5/20 in immediately post surgery and 14, 7/20 at last follow-up (p=0.2).
- These results lead to the conclusion that it is difficult to achieve an improvement of bone stock during a revision with an uncemented femoral stem, and, in a lot of cases, we have to fear secondary deterioration of the bone stock. It is thus better to define in detail the various types of bone

deficits to determine which path to be follow to avoid degradation of bone stock or to favor its regeneration when it has been altered by a loose implant (see Part V).

11.2.2 Bone Remodeling After Implantation of an Uncemented Femoral Stem

To designate all bone modifications that can occur in contact with an uncemented implant, with the exception of bone necrosis, we prefer the generic term "***bone remodeling***".

We propose a new classification of these modifications which are particularly ranked according to the difficulties that they can entail in the case of a new intervention. A decrease of bone density, especially if associated with a decrease of the thickness of the cortices, increases the difficulty of a new intervention; on the other hand, cortical thickening does not constitute a real danger.

11.2.2.1 Classification

Table 11.4 Classification of bone remodeling

St.0: No bone modifications
St.1: Thickening of cortices in 3 and/or 5; thickness id or decrease +/– in 2 and/or 6 and no modifications of bone density (Fig. 11.7)
St.2: Decrease of bone density =/<2 zones and thickness of cortices unchanged (Fig. 11.8)
St.3: Decrease of bone density > in 2 zones and thickness of cortices unchanged (Fig. 11.9)
St.4: Decrease of bone density > in 2 zones and thickness of cortices decreased (Fig. 11.10)

NB: A decrease of bone density on top of a cortical thickening is classified stage 2 or, more rarely, stage 3.

Bone remodeling that can occur in the contact of an uncemented implant are evaluated by taking the Gruen zones as a reference: cortical thickening is evaluated according to its localization, and a decrease in bone density according to its extent and the cortical thickness that can have decreased or not.

This classification does not include the bone regeneration which must be considered as being normal in the context of revision and only a significant decrease of the osseous density is taken account.

In our series of 150 patients, bone remodeling was evaluated as follows: stage 0: 93 cases; stage 1: 6 cases; stage 2: 19 cases; stage 3: 19 cases; stage 4: 13 cases.

11.3 Discussion

- Firstly, in revision with an uncemented femoral stem, the method proposed by Engh et al. [20] to evaluate the overall secondary bone stock is neither adapted nor sufficient. Not adapted, because the importance given to Gruen zone 7 seems disproportionate as it is often absent or limited to a small distance in revision surgery. Insufficient especially, because this method does not allow evaluation of every modification that bone can be exposed to when in contact with an uncemented femoral stem. We think in particular of the various aspects of degradation of bone stock (see below: bone remodeling and results of secondary bone stock); or, on the contrary, bone regeneration, in the case of a revision. The method proposed by Boisgard et al. [21] to evaluate bone regeneration in revisions is interesting, but it does not take into account all types of bone changes that can have an influence on the long-term clinical results or in the hypothesis of an iterative surgery what increases the risks of a too favorable interpretation.
- Secondly, in revision, using the preoperative radiological classification of Della Valle and Paprosky [10] or the

SOFCOT classification [12] as a reference to evaluate the bone stock, is a cause of error because the osseous damages are often underestimated and these classifications do not take into account degradation of bone stock that could be caused by the surgeon during intervention ! A radiographic evaluation performed immediately after surgery always constitutes a safer reference for evaluation of secondary preservation, regeneration or degradation of bone stock, or for measuring the possible impact of an initial degradation of the bone stock on the secondary bone stock.

11.3.1 Bone Remodeling and Results of Secondary Bone Stock (n 150)

- Bone remodeling et secondary bone stock are significantly dependent (p<0.0001): bone remodeling classified as stage 3 or 4 (n 50) was noted in 64% of the cases rated as having average/poor secondary bone stock (32 vs 50 cases). A decrease of bone density, often accompanied by a decrease of the cortical thickness, is thus the main reason for poor radiographic results of the secondary bone stock in our series of patients.

Table 11.5 Bone remodeling and secondary bone stock

Bone remodeling Second. bone stock	Stage 0 (n 93)	Stage 1 (n 6)	Stage 2 (n 19)	Stage 3 (n 19)	Stage 4 (n 13)
Very good (n 66)	58	4	4	/	/
Good (n 34)	23	2	9	/	/
Average (n 27)	8	/	4	12	3
Poor (n 23)	4	/	2	7	10

- We found only six cases of bone remodeling stage 1 in the form of cortical thickening in zones 3 and/or 5, and none of these patients presented a hypotrophy of the overlying proximal femur. In these cases, we suspect a deviation of load transmission to the distal femur. Such cortical hypertrophies occur mostly in situations of good bone quality (absence of osteoporosis) and they probably deserve a special status, as they usually have moderate or no functional consequences (see following table). Their presence does not hinder a possible new intervention under favorable conditions.

11.3.2 Bone Remodeling and Clinical Results According to Harris (n 150)

Taking the difference between the preoperative and postoperative clinical results as a reference, as proposed by Harris, the mean deviation for patients stage 0 (n=93) is +35.8 versus +31.6, average of the results for the patients stage 3 and

4 (*n=32*). This represents a significant degradation (p<0.0001); the same is true – but this time in terms of an improvement – for patients stage 1 (cortical thickening), where mean deviation is +45.9 versus +35.8 for patients with no cortical modifications

Table 11.6 Bone remodeling and clinical results

Bone remodeling Clinical results (HHS)	Stage 0 (*n 93*)	Stage 1 (*n 6*)	Stage 2 (*n 19*)	Stage 3 (*n 19*)	Stage 4 (*n 13*)
Preoperative	47.1	45.1	48.3	49	43.2
Postoperative	82.9	91	84.3	80.9	74.5
Deviations	+35.8	+45.9	+36	+31.9	+31.3

Contrary to Paprosky's opinion [25] for revision stems, and Abadie's et al. [26] or Bugbee's et al. [27] for primary stems, a decrease of bone density, sometimes associated with cortical atrophy, is not totally without clinical repercussions. This is evidenced by the 32 cases stage 3 and 4 of our series that show less good clinical results. Significantly this population consists of a majority of women (81% vs. 19% men) (p<0.001) compared with 39% vs. 61% for the 93 patients who present no bone remodeling. The higher prevalence of women to be subject to such an event was already reported for both, uncemented [27, 28] and cemented implants [26].

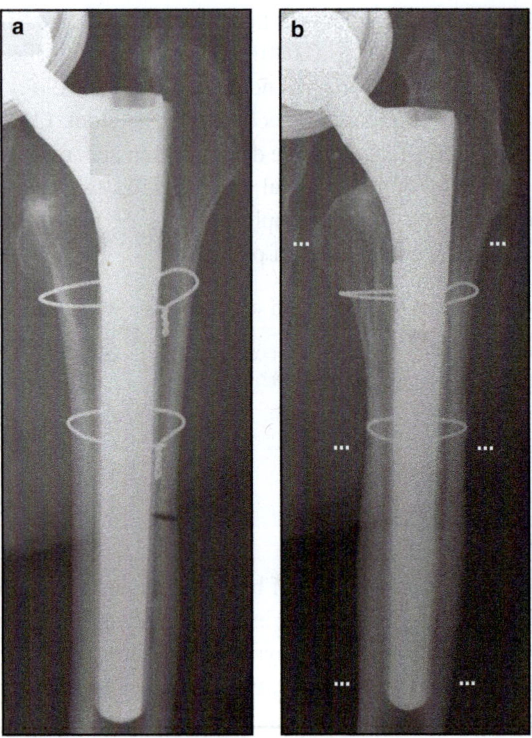

Fig. 11.7 Bone remodeling: stage 1. A 55-year-old female patient, femoral flap and short diaphyseal fixation, the medial cortex is not in contact with the implant (**a**). Results at 6 years: cortical hypertrophy in Gruen zones 3 and 5, no major modifications of the proximal femur. Bone stock, before: 18/20; after: good+ at 16/20 (**b**)

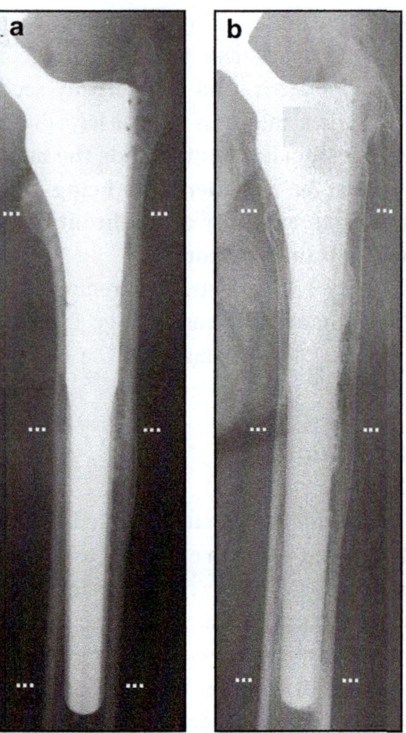

Fig. 11.8 Bone remodeling: stage 2. A 75-year-old female patient. Endofemoral approach and implantation of a short revision stem in combination with endomedullary bone graft and HA granules (**a**). Results at 7 years: significant decrease of the density of the cortices in zones 2 and 6. No diminution of thickness of cortices. Bone stock, before: 16/20; after: average at 10/20 (**b**)

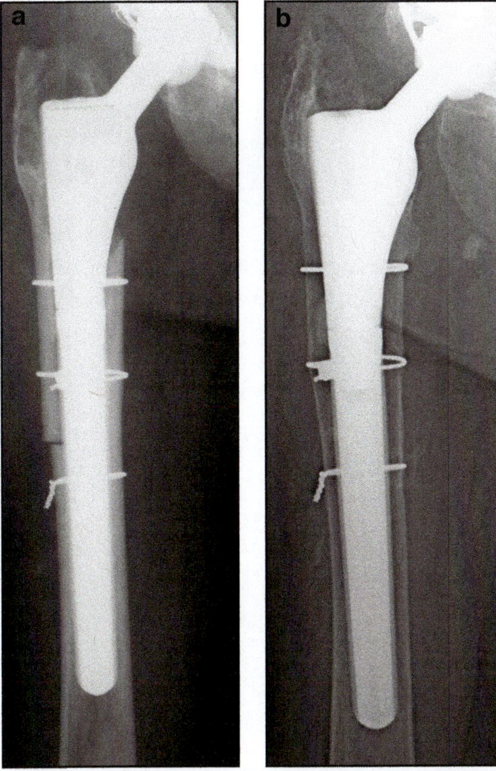

Fig. 11.9 Bone remodeling: stage 3. A 63-year-old female patient. Transfemoral approach and implantation of a short revision stem (**a**). Results at 11 years: significant decrease of the density of the cortices in zones 2, 3, 5 and 6 without diminution of thickness of cortices. Bone stock, before: 14/20; after: poor at 6/20 (**b**)

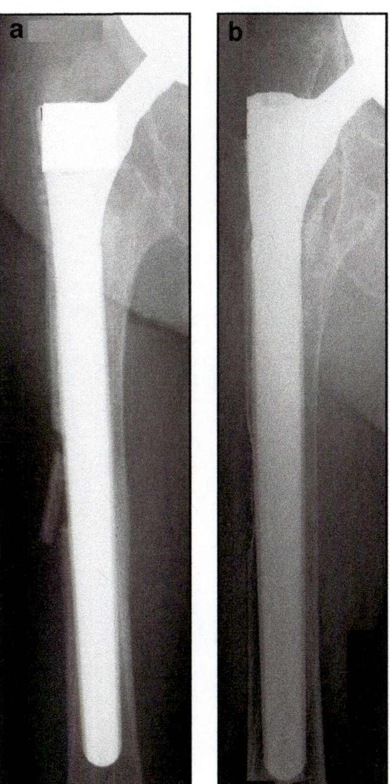

Fig. 11.10 Bone remodeling: stage 4. A 70-year-old female patient. Endofemoral approach + femoral window, implantation of a long stem with diameter 20 mm. Adding of HA granules (**a**). Results at 10 years: diminution of bone density with atrophy of the lateral cortex and necrosis of the femoral window and of the greater trochanter. Bone stock, before: 8/20; after: poor at 0/20 (**b**)

Evaluation of Osseointegration and Secondary Stability

The score proposed by Engh et al. [18] in 1990 for the radiographic evaluation of osseointegration and secondary stability of uncemented femoral primary stems, is also used for uncemented femoral revision stems. Today, when evaluating their results, most authors still use this method which, however, does not allow precise evaluation of the quality (or type) of secondary stability. Above all, the evaluation criteria of this method are sometimes questionable or difficult to apply to all the different types of implants.

12.1 Method

The evaluation of osseointegration and secondary stability is based on an analysis of the bone/implant interface. Only a radiolucent line is taken into account, independent of its thickness and knowing that a strictly localized radiolucent line at the shoulder of the implant is not recorded.

This evaluation is done on two a/p radiographs that are taken at the latest follow-up (one classical and one negative). Two femoral zones are identified: the proximal femur corresponding to Gruen zones 1, 2 and 6 and the distal femur corresponding to zones 3 and 5. For these two femoral zones, the radiolucent line is, on the one hand, *quantified*, and, on the other hand, *qualified*.

- The radiolucent line is ***quantified*** at the level of every femoral zone (proximal and distal), depending on its extent, from 10 to 4 points: 10 points (no radiolucent line), 7 points (if =/<50%) or 4 points (if >50%). The total of the two zones leads to a score of osseointegration so-called "raw" score, which is calculated on 20 points with a distribution in four stages: very good (20); good (17); average (14); poor (11–8). This score is primarily used to study the factors that could influence the final results, and, possibly to compare the results with those of other authors.
- The so-called raw score is then ***qualified*** by a number 1, 2 or 3 for the proximal femur, and by a letter a, b or c for the distal femur. This makes it possible to define the type of secondary stability depending on the location of the radiolucent line. Depending on the type of secondary stability thus defined, a positive or negative weighting coefficient is added to obtain a so-called "weighted" final score. This is also done on the basis of 20 points with a distribution in four qualitative stages: very good (20–18); good (14); average (11); poor (5–8). For each qualitative stage a numerical mean is calculated.

Only the "weighted" score is taken into account to calculate the **G**lobal **R**adiographic **S**core and this score is also most frequently used for statistical studies or cross-analyses.

Table 12.1 Evaluation osseointegration and secondary stability

Evaluation radiolucent line			Osseointegration/secondary stability			
			Types of secondary stability	Raw Sc.	Weighting	Weighted Sc.
Proximal femur (Zones 1, 2 and 6)			**1a** Global stability 2+	20	0	**20**
1	○ St.1: lucent line absent	10	**1b** Global stability +	17	+1	**18**
2	○ St.2: lucent line =/<50%	7	**1c** Proximal stability +	14	0	**14**
3	○ St.3: lucent line >50%	4	**2a** Proximal stability −	17	−3	**14**
			2b Global stability +/−	14	0	**14**
Distal femur (Zones 3 et 5)			**2c** Fibrous stability +/−	11	0	**11**
a	○ St.1: lucent line absent	10	**3a** Dispheal stability	14	−3	**11**
b	○ St.2: lucent line =/<50%	7	**3b** Distal stability +	11	−3	**8**
c	○ St.3: lucent line >50%	4	**3c** Fibrous stab. +/ Loosening	8	−3	**5**
Osseointegration (raw sc.) **Total** /20 ○ very good (20); ○ good (17); ○ average (14); ○ poor (11–8)						
Secondary stab. (weighted sc.) **Total** /20 ○ very good (20–18); ○ good (14); ○ average (11); ○ poor (5–8)						

P. Le Béguec et al., *Uncemented Femoral Stems for Revision Surgery*,
DOI 10.1007/978-3-319-03614-4_12, © Springer International Publishing Switzerland 2015

12.2   Results

12.2.1 Results Osseointegration and Secondary Stabilities (*n 150*)

Table 12.2 Osseointegration and secondary stability (*n 150*) (*values in nb. and % and numerical*)

Results	Very good	Good	Average	Poor
Osseointegration	77	43	20	10
(*Raw score*)	(51%)	(29%)	(13%)	(7%)
Secondary stability	83	41	19	7
(*Weighted score*)	(55%)	(27%)	(13%)	(5%)
Secondary stability	**19.8**	**14**	**11**	**7.1**
(*Numerical score*)				

12.2.2 Raw and Weighted Score: Distribution of Patients

Table 12.3 Osseointegration and secondary stability: distribution patients (*n=150*)

Osseointegration (*raw sc.*) Sec. stability (*weighted sc.*)	Very good (*n 77*)	Good (*n 43*)	Average (*n 20*)	Poor (*n 10*)
Very good (*n 83*)	77	6	/	/
Good (*n 41*)	/	37	4	/
Average (*n 19*)	/	/	16	3
Poor (*n 7*)	/	/	/	7

The weighting of the "raw" score (osseointegration) had a positive effect on the results of 13 patients (9%) and finally, the numerical scores obtained decrease in progressive and logical manner, which tends to validate the method.

12.3   Types of Secondary Stability

Table 12. 4 Summary table of different types of secondary stability (*n 150*)

1a Global stability 2+	**VG** (20/20) n 77: no radiolucent line proximal and distal femur
1b Global stability +	**VG** (18/20) n 6: no radiolucent line proximal femur and =/<50% zones 3 and 5
1c Proximal stability +	**G** (14/20) n 0: no radiolucent line prox. femur but present >50% in zones 3, 5
2a Proximal stability −	**G** (14/20) n 37: radiolucent line zone 1 and <50% zones 2 and 6, none in distal femur
2b Global stability +/−	**G** (14/20) n 4: radiolucent line <50% prox. femur and zones 3 and 5
2c Fibrous stability+/−	**Av** (11/20) n 3: radiolucent line =/<50% prox. femur and =/>50% zones 3 and 5
3a Diaphaseal stability	**Av** (11/20) n 16: radiolucent line >50% proximal femur, but not in zones 3 and 5
3b Distal stability +	**P** (8/20) n 5: radiolucent line >50% proximal femur and =/<50% in zones 3 and 5
3c Fibrous + stab./Loosening	**P** (5/20) n 2: none or precarious osseointegration, deviation, subsidence

12.3.1 Secondary Stability: Very Good Results (*n 83*) (Final Rating 20–18)

These are cases that were qualified as having global stability 2+ (*n 77*) with a final score of 20/20 (Figs. 12.1 and 12.2). The patients with global stability + (*n 6*), with a final score of 18/20, were included in this category after weighting of +1 point because the radiolucency was not extensive, usually very fine, and, particularly, limited to the distal region of the femur. The proximal femur was perfectly osseointegrated (Fig. 12.3).

These two situations, which augur well for good long-term stability, do not always equate with good bone conditions. These cases can be accompanied by a loss of bone density.

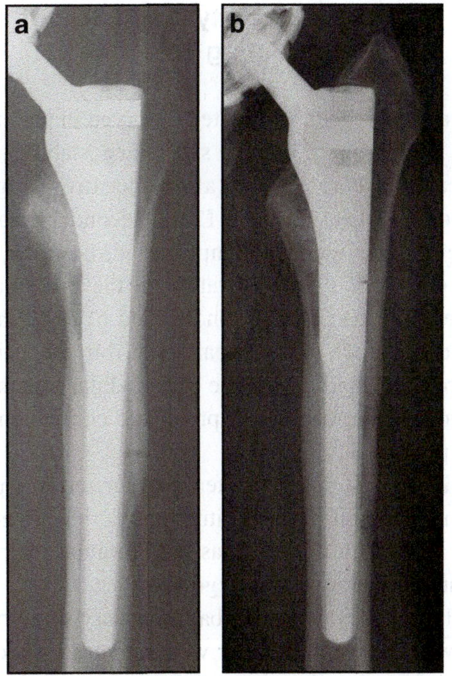

Fig. 12.1 A 27-year-old male patient, revision by endofemoral approach with a femoral window after a via falsa (**a**). At the 6-year follow-up, perfect osseointegration of the entire implant, secondary stability: global 2 +, very good 20/20 (**b**)

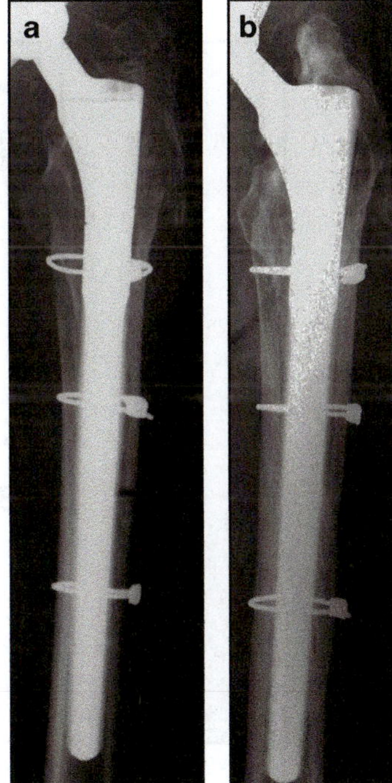

Fig. 12.2 A 77-year-old female patient, revision by transfemoral approach with a long revision stem (**a**). At the 6-year follow-up, good global osseointegration of the implant, slight decrease of the bone density in zones 3 and 6. Secondary stability: global 2+, very good 20/20 (**b**)

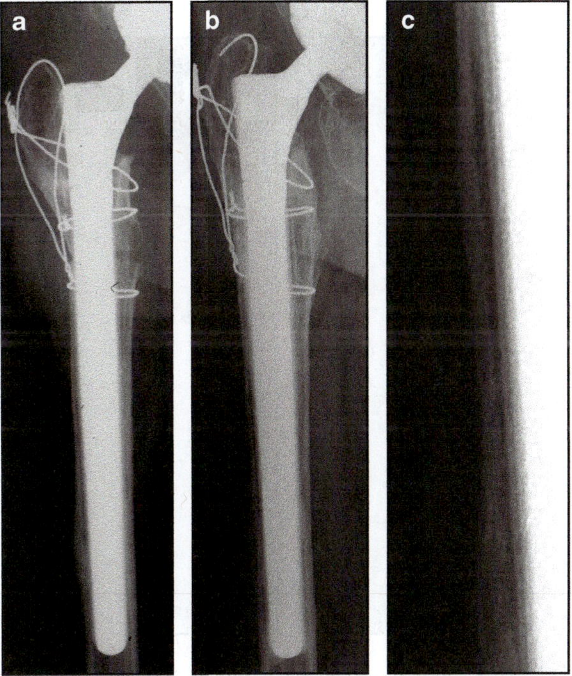

Fig. 12.3 69-year-old female patient, revision by an enlarged trochanterotomy + osteotomy of the medial cortex (**a**). At the 6-year follow-up, good proximal osseointegration (**b**), localized radiolucency localized in zone 3, at the level of the distal femur (**c**). Secondary stability: global +, very good 18/20 after weighting of +1 point

12.3.2 Secondary Stability: Good Results (*n 41*) (Final Rating 14)

- These good results were often observed in patients qualified as having proximal secondary stability – (*n 37*) with a final score of 14/20 after a negative weighting of −3 points (Figs. 12.4 and 12.5). Secondary stability in these patients was not compromised, however, a localized deficit of osseointegration in the proximal femur (zone 1 and partially in zones 2 and 6) can constitute a way of entrance for wear particles from the articulating components, and in the case of a modular prosthesis, the assembly zone of the two prosthetic components is not well protected.

  NB: Even if not encountered in our series, a proximal secondary stability + is a situation that has, in general, a good long-term prognosis as the proximal region of the femur is perfectly osseointegrated.

- For the cases evaluated global secondary stability ± (*n 4*), the two zones of the femur were affected by a deficit of osseointegration, but the radiolucency is =/<50% in the proximal and distal femur and the proximal portion of the implant (zone 1) is osseointegrated (Fig. 12.6).

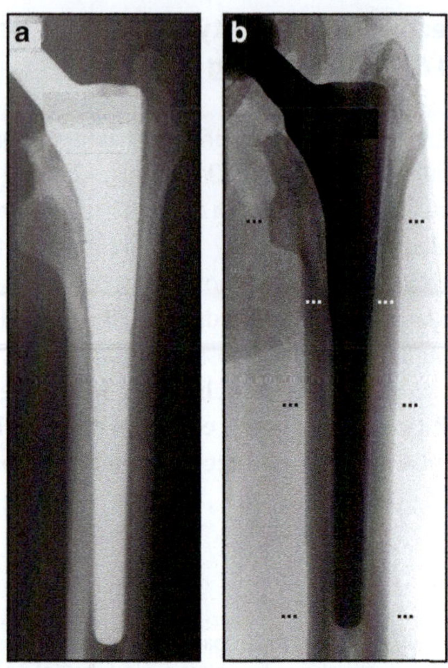

Fig. 12.4 A 60-year-old male patient, revision by endofemoral approach with a short stem (**a**). At the 6-year follow-up, deficit of osseointegration in the proximal femur </=50% in zones 2 and 6. Secondary stability: proximal −, good: 14/20 after weighting of −3 points of the raw score (**b**)

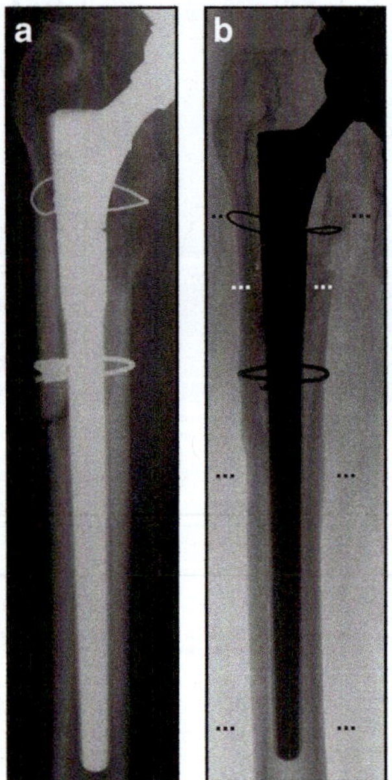

Fig. 12.5 A 70-year-old male patient, revision by transfemoral approach with a long stem (**a**). At the 5-year follow-up, lack of osseointegration </=50% proximal femur. Secondary stability: proximal −, good: 14/20 after weighting of −3 points of the raw score (**b**)

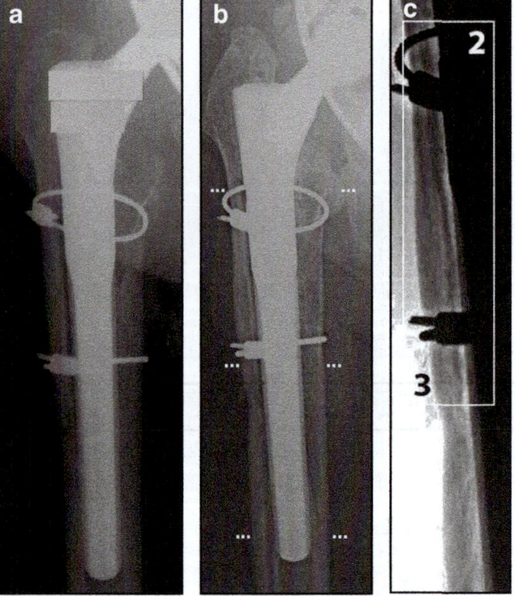

Fig. 12.6 A 61-year-old female patient, revision by transfemoral approach with a short stem (**a**). At the 9-year follow-up, deficit of osseointegration in zones 2 and 3, however, less than 50% in the proximal and distal femur. No radiolucencies in zone 1. Secondary stability: global ±, good: 14/20 (**b**). In the distal zone 3, spongialization of the endosteal bone which should not be confused with a radiolucency (**c**)

12.3.3 Secondary Stability: Average Results (*n 19*) (Final Rating 11)

- Distal stability (*n 16*) means a radiolucency >50% in the proximal femur and no radiolucency in zones 3 and 5 (Figs. 12.7 and 12.8). The "raw" score (14/20) was weighted negatively by −3 points because the radiolucency is proximal and is, in addition to its extent, often wide and sometimes progressive.
- When more than 50% of the implant surface destined for osseointegration is not integrated, the stability is defined as Fibrous +/− (Fig. 12.9). In these cases, (*n 3*), the prosthesis remains stable.

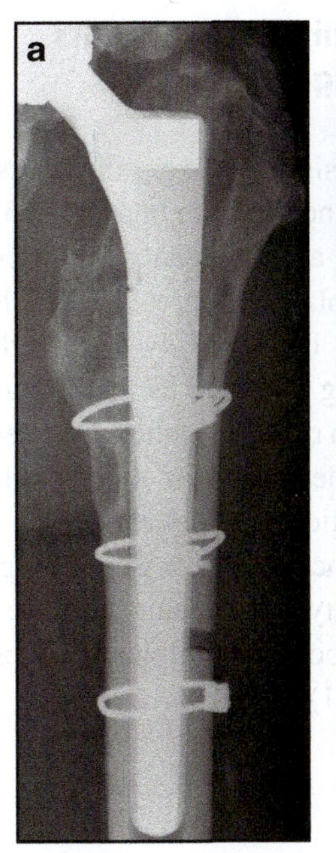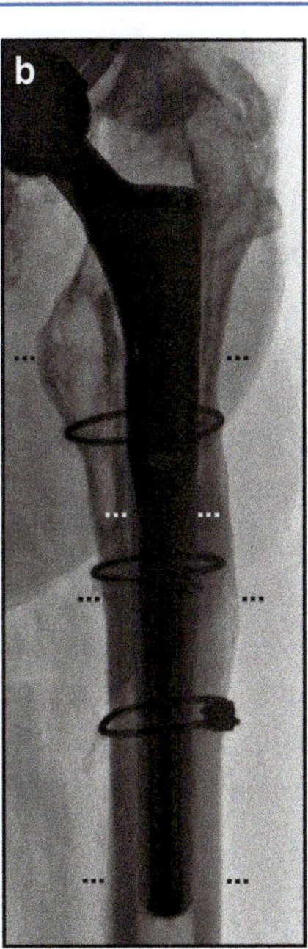

Fig. 12.7 A 70-year-old male patient, revision by transfemoral approach with a short stem (**a**). At the 13-year follow-up, radiolucency in the proximal femur in zones 1 and >50% in zones 2 and 6. Secondary stability: distal +, average: 11/20 after weighting −3 points (**b**). **NB**: Bordering line adjacent to radiolucency in zones 1 and 6

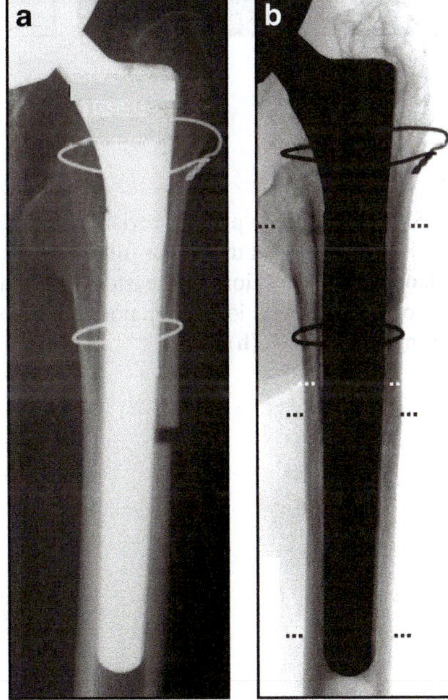

Fig. 12.8 A 74-year-old female patient, revision by transfemoral approach with a short stem (**a**). At the 3-year follow-up, radiolucency in the proximal femur zones 1 and >50% in zones 2 and 6. Secondary stability: distal +, average: 11/20 after weighting −3 points (**b**). **NB**: Radiolucency with a "bordering" line in zone 6

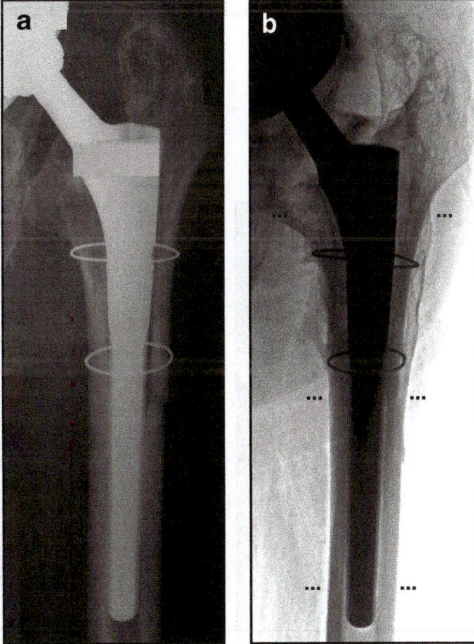

Fig. 12.9 A 72-year-old patient, revision by transfemoral approach with a short stem (**a**). At the 9-year follow-up, radiolucency ≤50% proximal and distal femur. Secondary stability: fibrous +/−, average: 11/20 (**b**)

12.3.4 Secondary Stability: Poor Results (*n 7*) (Final Rating 8–5)

- Distal stability + (*n 5*) designates a very distal osseointegration over a short distance (approximately 2–3 cm) in zones 3 and 5 as well as a radiolucent line, often large, present in most of the implantation area (Fig. 12.10). The initial raw score (11/20) is negatively weighted by −3 point. This is an alarming situation as there is a risk of sudden loosening during a routine rotational movement or of a fatigue fracture of the implant if it does not have a large diameter and the patient is overweight.
- Loosening (*n 2*) is characterized by various signs that indicate abnormal mobility of the femoral stem: varisation with a gap between bone and implant +, subsidence with bone plug (Fig. 12.11).

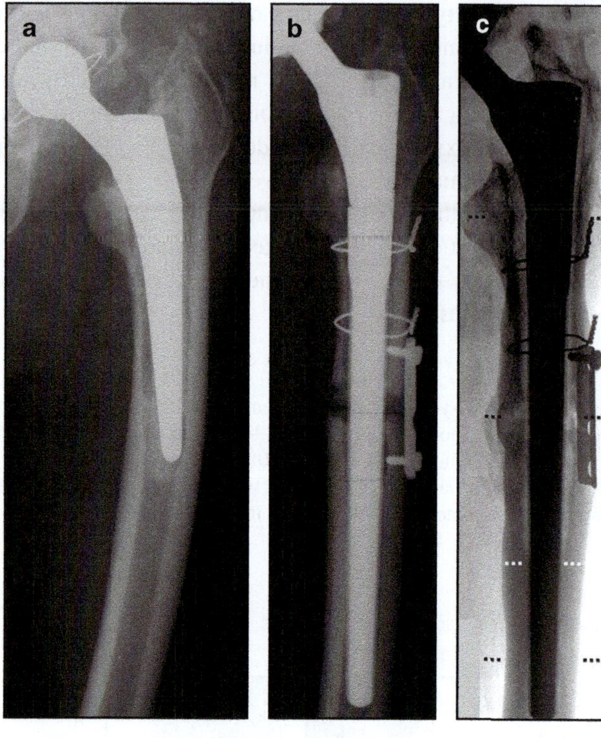

Fig. 12.10 A 75-year-old male patient, loosening of a cemented femoral stem in a femur with pronounced varus curvature (**a**). Revision by transfemoral approach with a long stem and an osteotomy of the medial cortex (**b**). At the 4-year follow-up, radiolucency in the proximal femur and #50% in the distal femur. Stability is only assured in the distal zone of the implant. Secondary stability: distal +, poor: 8/20 after negative weighting of −3 points (**c**)

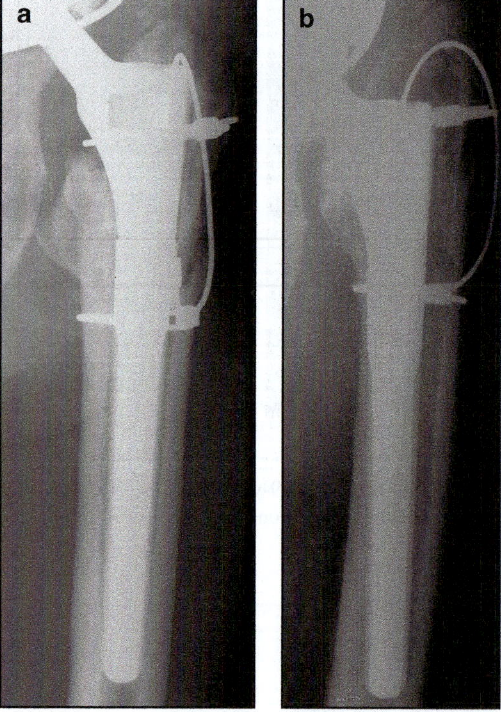

Fig. 12.11 A 67-year-old male patient, revision by trochanterotomy approach and a short stem (**a**). At the 7-year follow-up the gap between bone and implant (varus deviation of the stem) indicates abnormal mobility ++. Secondary stability: loosening, poor final score: 5/20 after negative weighting of −3 points (**b**)

12.4 Discussion

12.4.1 Criteria for Osseointegration

- A radiolucent line always indicates a gap between bone and implant that is filled with fibrous tissue, thus preventing the formation of bony bridges between cortex and implant. This criterion applies to all surfaces that can be osseointegrated; its absence is a sign of true osseointegration. Quantitative evaluation of the extent of a radiolucent line, however, is not sufficient, it must be qualified also. Its location needs to be assessed as well knowing that a perfect proximal osseointegration has a favorable prognosis, even if there is a deficit in the distal portion of the femur, and it does not have the same significance as an osseointegration limited to the distal zones 3 and 5. This finding justifies the introduction of a "weighted" score.
- When evaluating the stability of an implant, it is important to eliminate all criteria that do not clearly indicate a deficit of osseointegration.
  - This is the case of a so-called "reactive" line, which corresponds to a corticalization of the cancellous bone tissue at distance from the implant with bone tissue in direct contact with the implant. Such an image should not be confused with a "bordering" line that delimits a radiolucent line (Figs. 12.7 and 12.8).
  - Spongialization indicates a reduction of the density of the cortical bone in the contact area with the implant (Fig. 12.12). This radiographic appearance is not an equivalent of a radiolucency nor a sign of an osseointegration deficient. In the worst case, its presence can indicate a more precarious osseointegration. If it is located in the distal region, with perfect proximal osseointegration, such an image probably indicates that the zone of stabilization has become more proximal after a few years [4]. Such an evolution is rather reassuring and often an indication of a well designed implant. However, if a spongialization is located in the proximal region of the femur (zones 2 and 6), with cortical thickening in the distal region (zones 3 and 5), abnormal load transmission in the femur should be suspected.

Nb: For secondary subsidence and pedestal formation, criteria used by Engh for the evaluation of osseointegration and secondary stability, refer to Chap. 14.

12.4.2 Secondary Stability and Secondary Bone Stock (*n 150*)

No significant association between secondary stability (weighted score), as previously defined, and the value of secondary bone stock was found as: 76% of the patients rated as having average-poor secondary bone stock (i.e. 38 vs. 50 patients) were found to have very good-good secondary stability. On the other hand, 54% of the patients rated as having average-poor secondary stability (i.e. 14 vs. 26 patients) had a secondary bone capital that we evaluated as very good or good (p=0.1).

Table 12.5 Secondary stability and secondary bone stock

Secondary stability Secondary bone stock	Very good (*n 83*)	Good (*n 41*)	Average (*n 19*)	Poor (*n7*)
Very good (*n 66*)	45	15	4	2
Good (*n 34*)	15	11	7	1
Average (*n 27*)	13	8	4	2
Poor (*n 23*)	10	7	4	2

These results show that the two evaluations should be separated. Perfect osseointegration is not always a sign of good quality of the bone surrounding an implant, and a significant loss of bone density with cortical thinning (stress shielding stage 4 according to Engh) is often compatible with good osseointegration.

NB: For study of validity see Chap. 14: comparative elements with the Engh score.

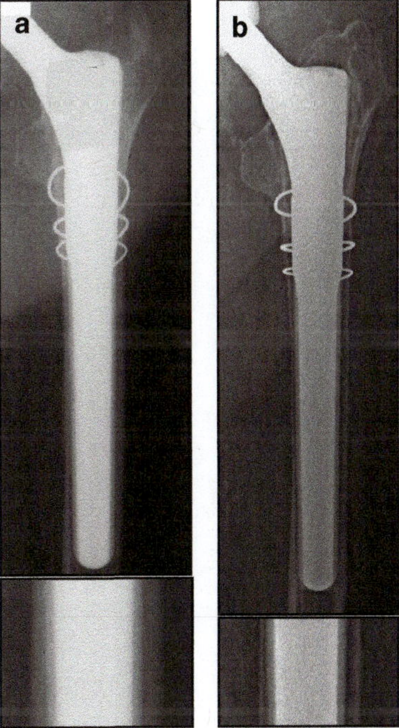

Fig. 12.12 A 63-year-old female patient. Osteoporotic femur and implantation of a short press-fit stem with a perfect bone/implant contact in zones 3 and 5 (*a1*) (**a**). At 10 years post surgery: secondary bone stock 2/20 because of major stress shielding that can be attributed to excessive stiffening of the bone/implant couple. Osseointegration rated as good at 14/20 (classification: proximal fixation -). Global Radiographic Score rated as poor: 10/20 (**b**). **NB**. Spongialization of the endosteal bone in zones 3 and 5 that must be distinguished from a radiolucent line (*b1*)

The **G**lobal **R**adiographic **S**core is a synthesis of the two evaluations: secondary bone stock and secondary stability (weighted score). These two evaluations have the same importance. Each of them is rated on a scale of 10 and the final result is based on 20 points with a distribution in four stages: very good (20); good (18–16–15); average (13–12); poor (=/<10).

A crossing between Global Radiographic Score and clinical results according to the Harris and a study of reproducibility have been performed.

13.1   Method

Table 13.1 Global evaluation secondary bone stock and secondary stability

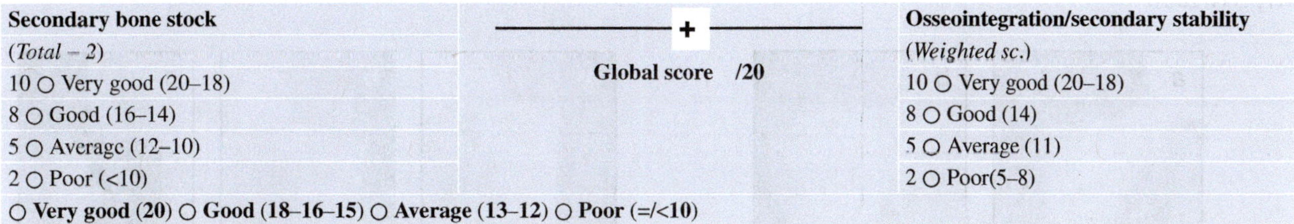

Secondary bone stock	+	Osseointegration/secondary stability
(*Total – 2*)		(*Weighted sc.*)
10 ○ Very good (20–18)	**Global score /20**	10 ○ Very good (20–18)
8 ○ Good (16–14)		8 ○ Good (14)
5 ○ Average (12–10)		5 ○ Average (11)
2 ○ Poor (<10)		2 ○ Poor(5–8)
○ **Very good (20)** ○ **Good (18–16–15)** ○ **Average (13–12)** ○ **Poor (=/<10)**		

NB. The marks attributed to the four stages of secondary bone stock and secondary stability, which yield the Global Radiographic Score, have been chosen in a way that clearly differentiates the four stages from each other – especially the cases rated as very good/good from those rated as average/poor.

The evaluations of the initial bone stock and of the osseointegration, "raw" score, are mainly used to examine the validity of the method and to study the factors that could have an impact on the final result.

- **Very good score** (rating 20) (Fig. 13.1). In this situation, there is no major deficience. Bone conditions are close to perfect, with at most a moderate defect (slight loss of bone density or of cortical thickness) in one zone of the femur. With regard to osseointegration, it is always perfect in the proximal femur, and if there is any deficit, it appears as a fine radiolucent line, relatively small and always located in the distal femur, which does not compromise the stability of the implant in the long term at all.

- **Good score** (rating 18–16–15) (Fig. 13.2). This stage includes more disparate situations with sometimes – in the best case – a situation close to a very good result (good +, score 18/20) and in the less good cases, close to an average result (good – , score 15/20).

- **Average score** (rating 13–12) (Fig. 13.3). In these cases, there is always a considerable or even major deficience, either of the bone stock or the secondary stability. Advanced forms of stress shielding (bone remodeling stages 3 or 4) are often found in this category of patients. These cases combine, on the one hand, a sharp decrease of bone density and cortical thickness (rating 2/10) with, on the other hand, perfect osseointegration of the implant (rating 10/10).

- **Poor score** (rating =/<10) (Fig. 13.4). This rating is not exclusively attributed to cases of loosening and abnormal mobility of the implant; situations with secondary stability qualified as distal + also fall into this category.

P. Le Béguec et al., *Uncemented Femoral Stems for Revision Surgery*,
DOI 10.1007/978-3-319-03614-4_13, © Springer International Publishing Switzerland 2015

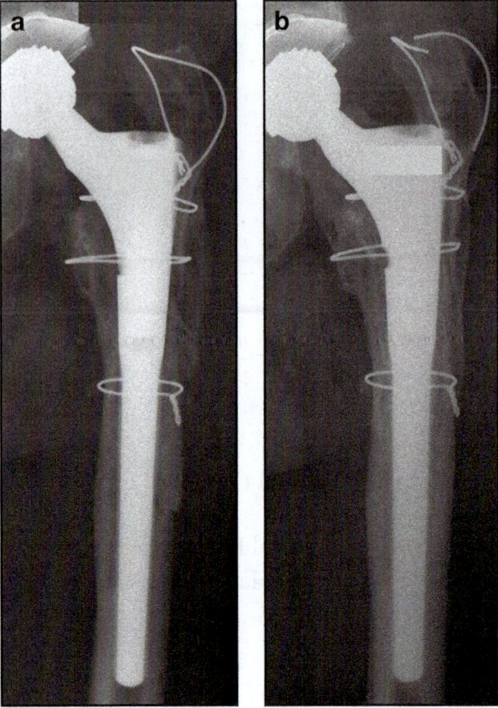

Fig. 13.1 A 89-year-old female patient. Revision by transfemoral approach and short stem (**a**). At the 4-year follow-up, perfect regeneration of bone stock without modification of the bone density: 20/20. Secondary stability: global 2+, 20/20 (**b**). Global Radiographic Score: very good 20/20

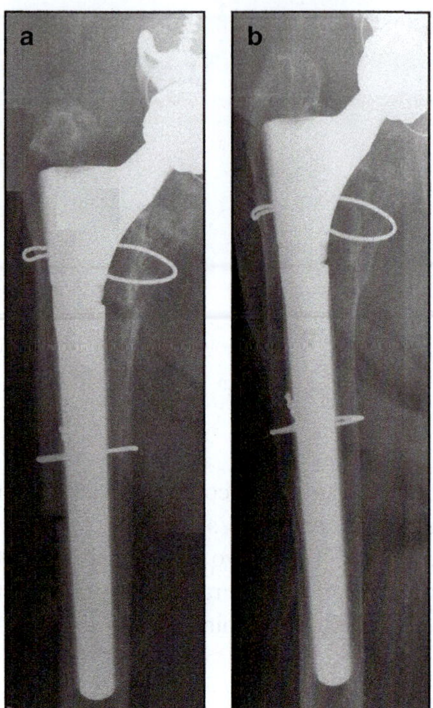

Fig. 13.3 A 78-year-old female patient. Transfemoral approach and implantation of a short revision stem (**a**). At the 5-year follow-up, sharp decrease of the density of the cortices, secondary bone stock: poor 8/20. On the other hand, perfect osseointegration and global secondary stability 2 + 20/20 (**b**). Global Radiographic Score: average 12/20

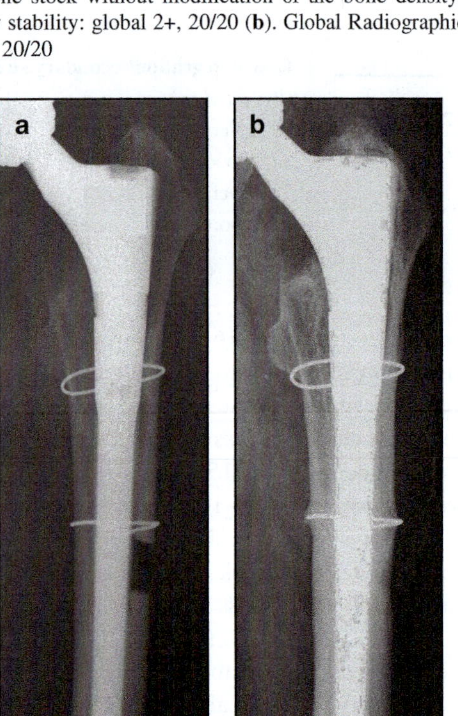

Fig. 13.2 A 67-year-old female patient. Revision by transfemoral approach and short stem, defect of the lateral cortex (gap of the flap) (**a**). At the 4-year follow-up, good filling of the bone defect, but decrease of the bone density (greater trochanter and zone 6): secondary bone stock good: 16/20. Radiolucent line =/<50% proximal femur proximal: secondary stability: proximal –, good 14/20 (**b**). Global Radiographic Score: good 16/20

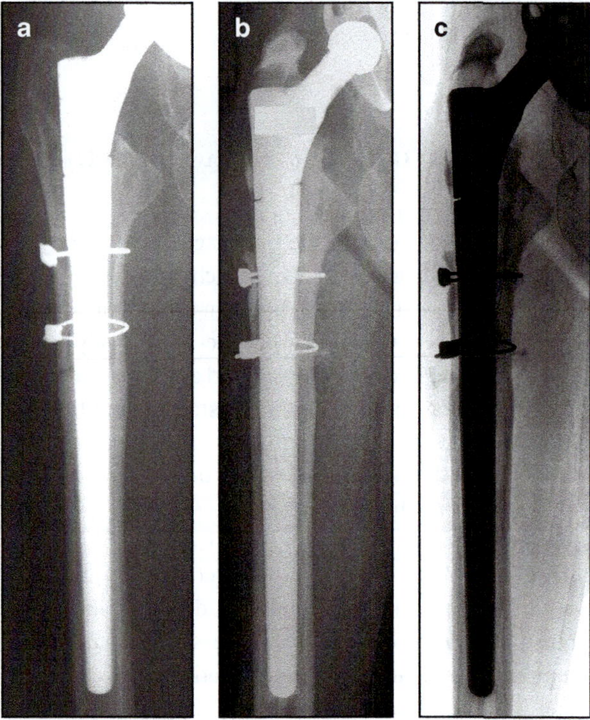

Fig. 13.4 A 71-year-old female patient. Transfemoral approach and implantation of a long revision stem (**a**). At the 4-year follow-up necrosis of the greater trochanter and +/− zone 2, reduced thickness in zone 3: secondary bone stock: poor 8/20. Radiolucent line >50% proximal femur: secondary stability distal + average 11/20 (**b**, **c**). Global Radiographic Score: poor 7/20

13.2 Results

The **G**lobal **R**adiographic **S**core was evaluated as very good: 44 times; good: 59 times; average: 27 times; poor: 20 times.

Table 13.2 The radiographic score

Radiographic scores	Very good	Good	Average	Poor
Secondary bone stock	66 (44%)	34 (23%)	27 (18%)	23 (15%)
Secondary stability (*weighted score*)	83 (55%)	41 (27%)	19 (13%)	7 (5%)
Global Radiographic Score	**44 (30%)**	**59 (40%)**	**27 (17%)**	**20 (13%)**

The evaluation of the bone stock and its integration into the global score had a negative impact on the **G**lobal **R**adiographic **S**core in the end. In comparison with the results obtained for the secondary stability (weighted score), there is a reduction of the percentage of very good results and an increase of cases rated as poor.

13.2.1 Clinical Results According to the Harris and Global Radiographic Score

The clinical score according to Harris was evaluated as follows: excellent in 53 patients (35%), very good in 46 patients (31%), good in 30 patients (20%), average in 15 patients (10%) and poor in 6 patients (4%).

The correlation between the clinical results and the Global Radiographic Score was assessed with a Kappa coefficient of –0.18, which reflects a very poor correlation.

Table 13.3 Clinic results and global radiographic score

Clinical score (HHS) / Global Rx score	Excellent (*n 53*)	Very good (*n 46*)	Good (*n 30*)	Average (*n 15*)	Poor (*n 6*)
Very good (*n 44*)	21	15	6	2	0
Good (*n 59*)	21	20	14	4	0
Average (*n 27*)	5	10	6	4	2
Poor (*n 20*)	6	1	4	5	4

Of the 129 patients that were rated as excellent, very good or good in their clinical results, 32 (25%) had an average or poor global radiographic score, and of the 21 evaluated as average-poor, 6 patients (29%) had a very good or good global radiographic score.

This poor correlation encourages the separation of the two evaluations. Combining the two evaluations into one score, as proposed by Kavanagh and Fitzgerald [29], does not mean that the final results will be good from both, the clinical and the radiographic perspective – especially if higher importance is given to the clinical results.

13.2.2 Study of Reproducibility

The *inter-observer* reproducibility of our method was done by two surgeons specialized in hip revision surgery (FB, OR) on the basis of 30 randomly selected postoperative radiographs. This same sample also served for the *intra-observer* reproducibility study, which was done 45 days later by the same surgeons who compared the results of the first and the second evaluation.

13.2.2.1 Inter-observer Reproducibility

In numerical scores: the intra-class correlation coefficient was globally good for the global score (ICC=0.8 with CI [0.6–0.9]), less good for the secondary bone stock (ICC=0.6 with CI [0.3–0.8]) and even less good for osseointegration (ICC=0.5 with CI [0.2–0.7]).

In categorized scores (VG/G/Av/P): for the global score, the weighted Kappa index was evaluated as 0.5 with CI [0.3–0.8] which demonstrates an average concordance. For the secondary bone stock, the index was 0.6 with CI [0.4–0.7], which indicates a rather good concordance; and for secondary stability, the weighted Kappa index was 0.4 with CI [0.1–0.7], which indicates a rather poor concordance.

13.2.2.2 Intra-observer Reproducibility (Tables Below)

For the global score, the intra-class correlation coefficient in numerical scores was very good; it was good according to the weighted Kappa index in categorized scores.

When referring to the two evaluations that make up the global score, we note that the reproducibility tests are globally less good for secondary stability (weighted score).

Table 13.4 Intra-observer reproducibility (*numerical scores*)

Intra-class correlation coefficient	Observer 1	Observer 2
Secondary bone stock	0.8 CI (0.7–0.9)	0.9 CI (0.91–0.98)
Secondary stability (*weighted score*)	0.5 CI (0.1–0.7)	0.7 CI (0.5–0.8)
Global Radiographic Score	**0.8 CI (0.6–0.9)**	**0.9 CI (0.7–0.9)**

Table 13.5 Intra-observer reproductibility (*categorized scores*)

Kappa index	Observer 1	Observer 2
Secondary bone stock	0.7 CI (0.4–0.9)	0.9 CI (0.8–0.99)
Secondary stability (*weighted score*)	0.6 CI (0.3–0.9)	0.6 CI (0.4–0.9)
Global Radiographic Score	**0.7 CI (0.5–0.9)**	**0.8 CI (0.6–0.9)**

In summary: The reproducibility of the proposed method seems satisfactory and the numerical value of a score makes it possible to better express a difference which may not appear obvious when the result is indicated in qualitative (or categorized) form.

The score developed by Engh et al. in 1990 [18], used by a vast majority of authors who report their radiographic results, only includes osseointegration and implant stability. The main objective of this score is to identify loosening, which is important but insufficient.

In addition to a validation study, which compares the results obtained with the Engh score to the score of secondary stability (weighted scores) and the Global Radiographic Score, we have made crossings to determine, particularly, the relevance of the criteria "secondary subsidence and pedestal" proposed by Engh to assess osseointegration and secondary stability of an uncemented femoral stem

14.1 Materials and Method

14.1.1 Validation Study

The method proposed by Engh was used to evaluate a consecutive series of 70 revision of the 150 patients assessed in this study and performed between September 1997 and September 1999. The results were rated as very good if the final score was higher than −10; good if it was between 0 and 10; average between 0 and 10 and poor if the score was inferior to −10. This same series of patients has been assessed according our method: secondary stability (weighted score) and the Global Radiographic Score, a synthesis of the scores for secondary stability and secondary bone stock.

With the help of the non-parametric correlation coefficient by Spearman, a validation study of our method was undertaken to compare the Engh score with the scores obtained according to our method. The study was done by two independent observers (FC, JB) on a cohort of 70 patients that were part of the 150 cases included in this study.

14.1.2 Crossings

On the basis of the entire cohort of 150 patients, several crossings were done between the secondary stability (weighted score) and the secondary subsidence of the stem as well as the presence of a pedestal. Another crossing was also done between secondary subsidence and the presence of a pedestal.

Two types of pedestals have been identified: partial, if only one cortex is affected and complete, if both cortices are affected. Subsidence was evaluated on two a/p radiographs, one taken immediately after revision surgery and the other at the last follow-up. At the level of the femur, a cerclage wire or the middle of the lesser trochanter were taken as reference. At the level of the stem, the assembly zone of the two prosthetic components serves as a reference. These measures were taken with the EvalNet software (LeadTools®; LEAD Technologies, Inc, Charlotte, NC, USA).

P. Le Béguec et al., *Uncemented Femoral Stems for Revision Surgery*,
DOI 10.1007/978-3-319-03614-4_14, © Springer International Publishing Switzerland 2015

Table 14.1 Evaluation osseointegration and stability according to Engh

Fixation Osseointegration	Osteophilic zone	No radiolucencies 5	Radiolucency <50% 0	Radiolucency >50% −5
	Bony bridges	Yes 5	Indetermined 0	No −2.5
Stability	Smooth zone	No radiolucency 5	Not visible 0	Extensive radiol. −5
	Pedestal	No 2.5	Below stable stem 0	Below unstable stem −3.5
	Deterioration interface	Unchanged 2.5	Indetermined 0	Radiolucency −2.5
	Migration	No 3	Indetermined 0	Yes −5
	Calcar	Atrophy 3	Indetermined 0	Hypertrophy −4
	Metal particle	No 1	Indetermined 0	Yes −5

Score	Osseointegration	Stability
>10	Yes	–
0 to 10	Suspected	Yes
0 to −10	No	Yes
<−10	No	No

14.1.3 Observations Regarding the Use of the Criteria from the Engh Score

This score uses criteria that are difficult to apply for a number of implants:

- An evaluation of the so-called "smooth" zone was not done, as there was no such zone in our case; on the other hand, the evaluation of the fixation (radiolucency and bony bridges) is relevant for the entire implant surface, which is, in the present case, osteophilic.
- The evaluation of the calcar was not taken into account as, in revision surgery, this zone of the femur is mostly absent during a revision.
- The presence or absence of metal particles was not assessed, as this criterion applies to a particular implant surface which was not the one of our study.
- Finally, "deterioration of the interface" was only taken into account when there was a deviation of the implant that created a significant gap between bone and implant (mostly because of varus position in the knowledge that the presence of a radiolucent line had already been taken into consideration before.

14.2   Results

Table 14.2 Comparison of results with Engh score (*n 70*)

Radiographic score	Very good	Good	Average	Poor
Secondary stability (*weighted score*)	40	20	7	3
Global radiographic sc.	23	29	10	8
Engh score	26	36	7	1

14.2.1 Validity Study

- The Spearman correlation coefficient, which compares the Global Radiographic Score with the Engh score, was considered average, yet significant ($r=0.57$). This is hardly surprising as this score also includes secondary bone stock, which is not the case in the Engh score.

Table 14.3 Validity study with the Engh score

Spearman correlation coef.	Global Rx score	Osseointegration (*raw score*)	Second, stability (*weighted score*)
Results (*n=70*)	**r=0.57** (IC 95%=0.38; 0.71)	**r=0.75** (IC 95%=0.62; 0.83)	**r=0.74** (IC 95%=0.61; 0.83)

- In contrast, the Spearman correlation coefficients can be considered as good and significant of a good correlation with the Engh score (p<0.0001) for osseointegration (raw score) (r=0.75) and secondary stability (weighted score) (r=0.74).

14.2.1.1 Comparison Between Secondary Stability Score and Engh Score (*n 70*)

(Correlation coefficient by Spearman considered as good [r=0.74; p<0.0001])

Table 14.4 Comparison secondary stability and Engh score

Second. stability (*weighted sc.*) Engh score	Very good (*n 40*)	Good (*n 20*)	Average (*n 7*)	Poor (*n 3*)
Very good (*n 26*)	25	1	/	/
Good (*n 36*)	15	16	5	/
Average (*n 7*)	/	3	2	2
Poor (*n 1*)	/	/	/	1

Patient distribution is coherent and the overall classification was respected. Only 11 patients (i.e. 16%) changed category: 3 patients (4%) were evaluated more strictly according to Engh and 8 patients (12%) were evaluated more.

14.2.1.2 Comparison Between Global Radiographic Score and Engh Score (*n 70*)

(Correlation coefficient by Spearman considered as average [r=0, 57; p<0.0001])

Table 14.5 Comparison global radiographic score and Engh score

Global Rx score Engh score	Very good (*n 23*)	Good (*n 29*)	Average (*n 10*)	Poor (*n 8*)
Very good (*n 26*)	15	10	1	/
Good (*n 36*)	8	17	6	5
Average (*n 7*)	/	2	3	2
Poor (*n 1*)	/	/	/	1

This study shows essentially the same ranking for the results assessed as very good and good. Only two cases rated as good according to the Global Radiographic Score were rated as average according to the Engh score. On the other hand, the results rated as average-poor showed a significant discrepancy: 8 cases with the Engh score versus 18 cases with the Global Rx Score, and, among the 18 patients rated as average-poor according to the Global Rx Score, 12 patients (67%) are rated as very

good-good according to the Engh score. This result confirms that integrating the parameter assessing secondary bone stock in the radiographic results worsens the final outcome!

14.2.2 Crossings

14.2.2.1 Secondary Stability and Secondary Subsidence (*n 150*)

The statistical analysis did not find a significant correlation between secondary stability (weighted score) and secondary subsidence (p=0.1).

Table 14.6 Secondary stability and subsidence

Secondary stability Secondary subsidence	Very good (*n 83*)	Good (*n 41*)	Average (*n 19*)	Poor (*n 7*)
0 mm (*n 80*)	43	25	9	3
1 to 4 mm (*n 41*)	26	9	4	2
5 to 10 mm (*n 17*)	9	3	5	0
>10 mm (*n 12*)	5	4	1	2

Among the 26 patients whose secondary stability was rated as average-poor, 18 patients (i.e. 69%) showed not significant secondary subsidence (>4 mm), and among the 29 patients who present a secondary subsidence ≥5 mm, 21 patients (i.e. 72%) were assessed as having very good-good secondary stability.

These results tend to prove that a secondary subsidence does not always indicate a deficit of osseointegration and stability, as suggested by Engh and Epinette.

If secondary migration in a cemented stem or in an uncemented self-locking stem can only occur in the case of true instability (and, in this case, a radiolucent line is often discernible), the same is not true for an uncemented stem with press-fit fixation. Such a concept makes secondary subsidence possible (Fig. 14.1). It is, furthermore, simply a sign of re-wedging, and has not negative impact on osseointegration or secondary stability [30].

14.2.2.2 Secondary Stability and Pedestal (*n 150*)

The statistical analysis did not find a significant correlation between secondary stability (weighted score) and pedestal (p=0.9).

Table 14.7 Secondary stability and pedestal

Secondary stability Pedestal	Very good (*n 83*)	Good (*n 41*)	Average (*n 19*)	Poor (*n 7*)
Absent (*n 99*)	53	29	13	4
Partial (*n 31*)	16	10	4	1
Complete (*n 20*)	14	2	2	2

Among the 51 patients with partial or complete pedestal, 30 patients (i.e. 59%) were rated as having very good secondary stability, and only 3 patients (6%) were rated as poor, Based on these findings, it is difficult to make this sign a criterion for instability.

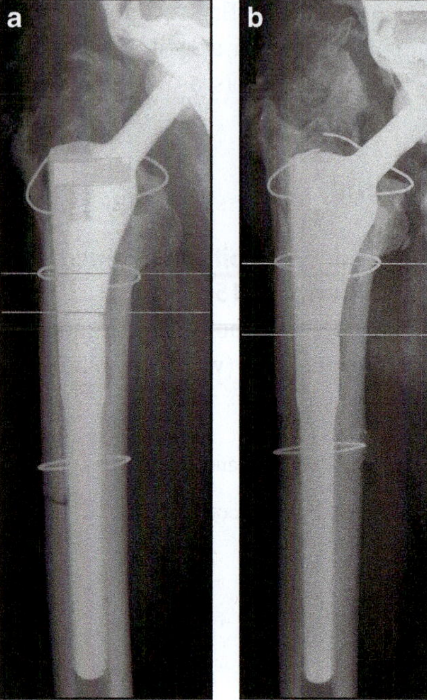

Fig. 14.1 71-year-old patient, revision by transfemoral approach and short stem (**a**). At the 4-year follow-up, perfect osseointegration, in spite of a secondary subsidence measured as 7 mm. Secondary stability global 2+, very good 20/20 (**b**)

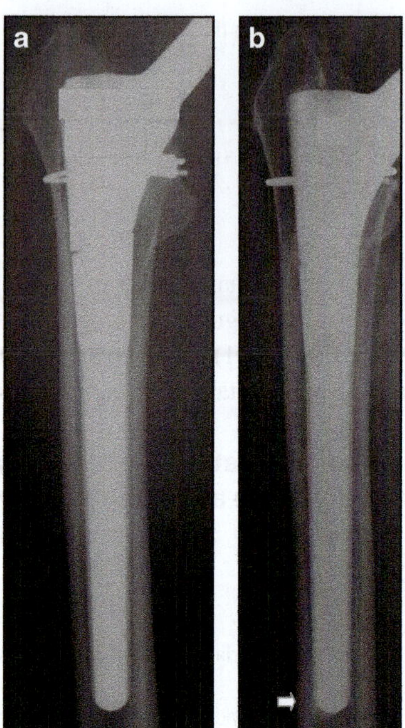

Fig. 14.2 65-year-old female patient, revision by endofemoral approach, distal tip of the implant in contact with the lateral cortex of the femur (**a**). At the 6-year follow-up not very significant secondary subsidence partial pedestal (**b**)

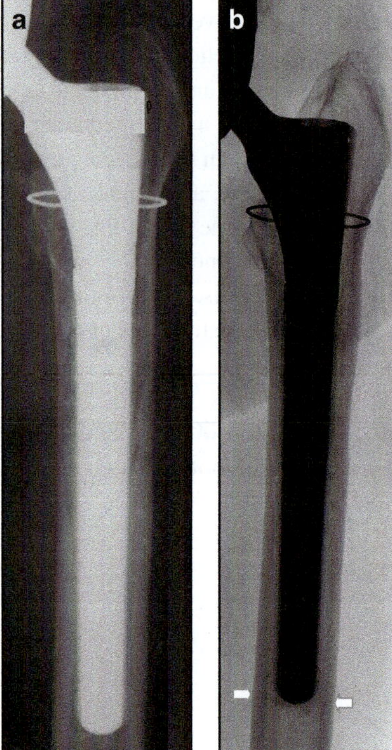

Fig. 14.3 69-year-old female patient, revision by endofemoral approach. Wide medullary canal, mean IC of 0.36, stem diameter 20 mm (**a**). At the 7-year follow-up, secondary subsidence $\neq 3$ mm, slight loss of the bone density of the lateral and medial cortices. Pedestal ± extensive (resulting from an anomaly in the load transmission?) (**b**)

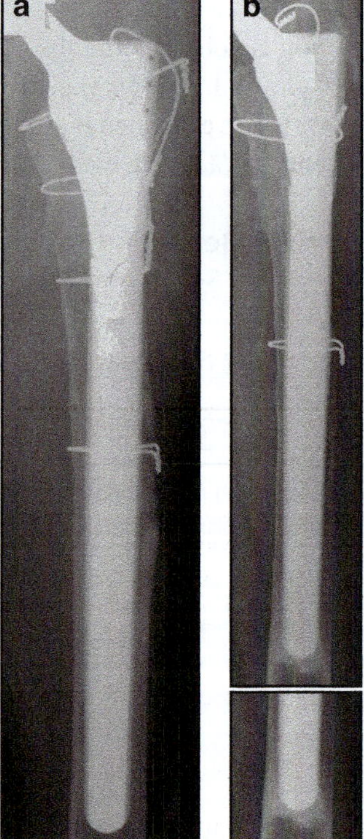

Fig. 14.4 71-year-old female patient, iterative loosening, osteoporotic femur. Revision by trochantero-diaphyseal flap, diaphyseal primary stability with a long stem of large diameter, cortical defect in zone 2 (**a**). At the 8-year follow-up, no bone regeneration in zone 2 and marked loss of bone density in the entire femur with cortical thinning in zones 3 and 5; poor secondary bone stock: 0/20. Complete pedestal, probably due to significant stiffening of the bone/implant couple and at the origin of an abrupt break in the transmission of the femoral constraints (**b**)

14.2.2.3 Pedestal and Secondary Subsidence (n 150)

Arguing that a pedestal could be an indirect sign of instability because it could be a sign of secondary subsidence, which Engh considers in itself as a sign of instability, is difficult to maintain based on this statistical analysis that did not find a significant correlation between secondary subsidence and the presence of a pedestal (p = 0.4).

Table 14.8 Pedestal and secondary subsidence

Pedestal	Partial	Complete
Secondary subsidence	(n 31)	(n 20)
0 mm (n 80)	14	10
1 à 4 mm (n 41)	11	4
5 à 10 mm (n 17)	4	5
> à 10 mm (n 12)	2	1

If it is only partial (Fig. 14.2), a pedestal can result from a simple conflict between the implant and one of the cortices. When it can be called "unstable", i.e. associated with a radiolucent line, it can result from an implant that cannot be osseointegrated in the distal zone (smooth distal tip) or indicates an instability of the implant and, in this case, the pedestal is often complete and/or a varus position of the implant can be observed.

A complete pedestal and a stable prosthesis (Figs. 14.3 and 14.4) could be attributed to excessive stiffening of the bone/implant couple, at the origin of an abrupt break in the transmission of the femoral constraints, especially if the femur is osteoporotic.

In Summary: Some of the criteria proposed by Engh cannot be used in all situations (presence metal particles, evaluation of a smooth prosthetic zone or modifications of the calcar in a revision). Others cannot be specifically attributed to instability (secondary subsidence or presence of a pedestal) and are therefore not essential for the evaluation of osseointegration and secondary stability of an uncemented implant.

Furthermore, the results of the secondary stability score (weighted score) as we have defined it, do not differ much from those obtained with the Engh score. Thus, 82% of the patients evaluated with our method (see table page 87) were rated as very good or good, i.e. the same figure as that given by Paprosky also of 82% [25] and very close to the figure of 81% given by Korovessis [31]; the two authors used the Engh score that includes secondary subsidence and pedestal formation in their evaluation method for evaluating osseointegration and secondary stability.

When proposing a new method for radiographic evaluation, one needs to be sufficiently precise without being too suggestive to leave a sufficient margin of maneuver to the user. This balance is difficult to find. If avoiding an accumulation of too many evaluation criteria can make a method easier to apply, it may also leave the assessor too much liberty.

Independent of which score is used, a good understanding of the method is the main criterion to allow its dissemination. The good results that we have obtained in our reproducibility seem to prove that the **G**lobal **R**adiographic **S**core that we have developed (see summary table: Appendix 1) is comprehensible and easy to use.

The Global Radiographic Score attempts to reflect exactly the behavior of the femoral bone around an implant and the capacity of an uncemented implant to integrate into the surrounding bone.

1. The quality of bone surrounding an uncemented implant (density and cortical thickness) should be carefully analyzed because a new intervention could always be possible. In the case of a revision, the evaluation of the secondary bone stock is also a necessity because the bone stock is often damaged in the beginning.
2. The evaluation of osseointegration should not be limited to the diagnosis of loosening. The quality of osseointegration (type of secondary stability) should also be carefully assessed. A deficit of proximal osseointegration does not bode well for the long term, especially if it has a tendency to move farther distally; in contrast, perfect proximal osseointegration of the implant is often a sign of perfect adaptation. The prognosis is thus good, especially if the surrounding bone has preserved a normal texture.

Part V

Evaluation of the Radiographic Results – Why?

Three objectives:

1. Report on the learning curve and its teachings.

2. Analysis of the factors that could have an impact on the radiographic results.
   - Different types of primary stability.
   - Degree of osteoporosis or bone condition.
   - Extent of the initial degradation of the bone stock.

3. Qualitative and numerical assessment of the radiographic results.

The learning curve is often used to explain a failure, yet rarely to improve the results. However, a critical review of failures or complications – inevitable in the beginning – is instructive. If such incidents occur with the designing surgeon, it is very likely that all users will be exposed to the same risks if they are not duly informed of the requirements imposed by a method.

The role of an author should not be limited to the proclamation of good results. Based on his experience and his own failures, he should provide guidance on how to obtain the best possible results. Everyone should benefit from the experience of everyone else!

15.1 Strategical Choices

In a retrospective study of 150 consecutive revisions of total hip prostheses, performed between April 1996 and December 2000 (142 patients), 2 chronological groups of 75 patients (groups 1 and 2) were identified to assess the evolution of the strategic choices and the previously defined results.

15.1.1 Femoral Approaches

At the start of the experiment (group 1), an endofemoral approach (or trochanterotomy) and a trochantero-diaphyseal flap were performed in approximately the same number of cases. In contrast, during the second period of the exercise (group 2), the endofemoral approach was abandoned in favor of a trochantero-diaphyseal flap that was performed in the vast majority of cases.

Table 15.1 Evolution of femoral approaches

	Global series (n 150) 04-96/12-00	Group 1 (n 75) 04-96/05-98	Group 2 (n 75) 05-98/12-00
Femoral approach			
Endofemoral	47 (31%)	40 (53%)	7 (9%)
Femoral flap	103 (69%)	35 (47%)	68 (91%)

A femoral window was done 13 times, mainly to excise a cement plug when an endofemoral approach had been chosen.

In 25% of the cases, an osteotomy of the medial cortex was associated with a lateral trochantero-diaphyseal flap. This was done essentially the same number of times in both patient groups.

15.1.2 Different Types of Primary Stability

The frequent use of a trochantero-diaphyseal flap in group 2 deprived us of the possibility to seek proximal or global stability (8% versus 32% of the cases in group 1) and is the reason for the diaphyseal primary stability achieved in 67% of the cases.

Table 15.2 Evolution of types of primary stability

	Global series (n 150) 04-96/12-00	Group 1 (n 75) 04-96/05-98	Group 2 (n 75) 05-98/12-00
Types primary stability			
Proximal	13 (9%)	12 (16%)	1 (1%)
Global	17 (11%)	12 (16%)	5 (7%)
Diaphyseal short	49 (33%)	8 (11%)	41 (55%)
Diaphyseal long	33 (22%)	24 (32%)	9 (12%)
3-points	38 (25%)	19 (25%)	19 (25%)

NB: Short diaphyseal stability = stem L. <250 mm and long diaphyseal stability = stem L. >250 mm

It may be interesting to note that a 3-point support was achieved at the same rate (25%) in the two patient groups, which means that the use of a femoral flap did not reduce this risk.

15.1.3 Length of the Implant

The preferred choice of a femoral approach by means of a trochantero-diaphyseal flap had the (paradoxal!) effect of a more frequent use of a short stem (height of metaphyseal part + length of diaphyseal part) i.e. a length of <200 mm:

P. Le Béguec et al., *Uncemented Femoral Stems for Revision Surgery*,
DOI 10.1007/978-3-319-03614-4_15, © Springer International Publishing Switzerland 2015

5% of the patients in group 1 versus 36% of the patients in group 2. In parallel, the number of stems with a length of >250 mm decreased: 56% of the patients in group 1 versus 21% of the patients in group 2. About the same number of medium-length stems (200–250 mm) were implanted in the two patient groups.

Table 15.3 Evolution of length of implants

	Global series (*n 150*)	Group 1 (*n 75*)	Group 2 (*n 75*)
Length of implant	04-96/12-00	04-96/05-98	05-98/12-00
<200 mm	31 (21%)	4 (5%)	27 (36%)
200–250 mm	61 (41%)	29 (39%)	32 (43%)
>250 mm	58 (38%)	42 (56%)	16 (21%)

15.2 Evolution of the Radiographic Scores

- Firstly, it is worth recalling the negative impact of taking the secondary bone stock into consideration when establishing the **R**adiographic **G**lobal **S**core. To improve the global result (i.e. reduce the number of poor results) the greatest potential for improvement is in the bone stock.
- Secondly, a marked improvement of the **G**lobal **R**adiographic **S**core should be noted in the patients of group 2 (p=0.02), which is due to an increase of the number of very good results (15 patients in group 1 versus 29 patients in group 2), associated with a decrease of the poor results (15 patients in group 1 versus 5 patients in group 2). The better results in group 2 are primarily due to a significant improvement of the results for secondary bone stock (p=0.02), with a marked decrease of

poor results (5 patients versus 18 patients in group 1); it was not possible to find a statistically significant improvement of the secondary stability (weighted score) (p=0.4).

15.3 Conclusions

1. Every author encounters difficulties during the different steps of developing a strategy or a surgical technique. The notion of a learning curve is a reality, and the role of an author is to provide every surgeon with the means to avoid errors that can occur in the beginning of an experience.
2. At first sight, the better results of the patients in group 2 could indicate that there is a correlation between the strategic choice, the quality of a surgical procedure and the final result. This is possible, however, it must also be noted that the initial bone stock is less affected in group 2 (0 cases rated as poor in group 2 versus 8 cases in group 1), and the number of cases with an osteoporosis rated as poor is smaller (2 cases in group 2 versus 16 in group 1). Thus, one would think that these two factors can also play a role, especially in the regeneration or the preservation of bone stock.
3. In the end, the following three events can have an impact on a radiographic result:
   - **The type of primary stability**, good reflection of the strategic choice and the surgical technique adopted by the surgeon.
   - **The degree of osteoporosis**, good reflection of the "bone condition" of the patient.
   - **The value of the initial bone stock** (immediately post-surgery), good reflection of the bone defects caused by loosening (and/or the surgeon!).

Table 15.4 Evolution of the radiographic scores

	Global series (*n 150*) 04-96/12-00				Group 1 (*n 75*) 04-96/05-98				Group (*n 75*) 05-98/12-00			
Radiographic scores	VG	G	Av	P	VG	G	Av	P	VG	G	Av	P
Secondary bone stock	66	34	27	23	29	14	14	18	37	20	13	5
Secondary stability (*weighted sc.*)	83	41	19	7	38	22	10	5	45	19	9	2
Global Radiographic Score	44	59	27	20	15	31	14	15	29	28	13	5

Different Types of Primary Stability and their Impact on the Radiographic Results (Bone Stock and Secondary Stability)

16

When an uncemented implant has been chosen, the type of primary stability achieved at the end of the surgery can have an impact – favorable or unfavorable – on the secondary bone stock and/or the secondary stability. This is also the only moment when the surgeon can directly influence one or several factors that could have a real impact on the final radiographic result.

16.1 The Different Types of Primary Stability

With an uncemented implant, it is easy to identify the zone of the femur where the primary stability is located on a control radiograph taken immediately after surgery. In the case of "press-fit" or "fit and fill" concepts, it corresponds to the zone of the femur where there is an intimate contact between the cortex and the implant in the form of a surface. In the case of a self-locking stem, it is the zone of the femur where the locking takes place.

It is thus possible to identify different types of primary stability that can be proximal, global, diaphyseal (short or long) or by means of a 3-point contact if there is no surface contact between the bone and the implant.

16.1.1 Proximal Stability

In this case, the zone of primary stability is located in the proximal femur, most often in the metaphyseo-diaphyseal zone; there is no primary fixation in the diaphyseal region (no intimate bone/implant contact).

- The endofemoral approach is usual. This type of primary stability, most often achieved with stems intended for primary surgery, is also possible in revision surgery if the femur is straight in the a/p plane and if there is no significant bone defect (Fig. 16.1a).
- It is also possible to achieve proximal primary stability by making a flap if the cortices are of good quality, in perfect contact with the implant and if the osteosynthesis (cerclage) is efficient (Fig. 16.1b).

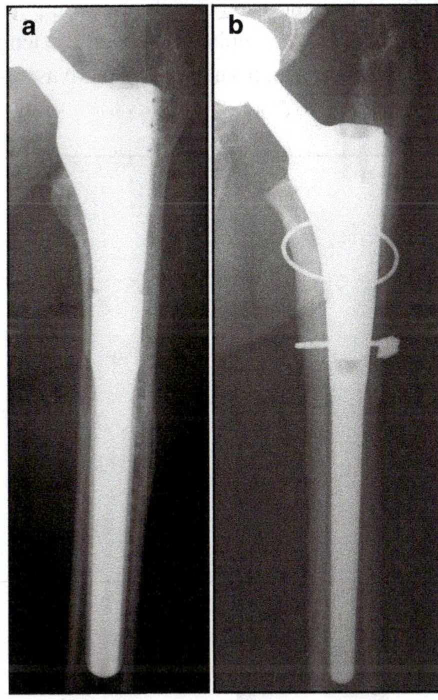

Fig. 16.1 Proximal primary stability by means of an endofemoral approach (**a**), after making a femoral flap (**b**)

P. Le Béguec et al., *Uncemented Femoral Stems for Revision Surgery*,
DOI 10.1007/978-3-319-03614-4_16, © Springer International Publishing Switzerland 2015

16.1.2 Diaphyseal Stability

The zone of primary stability can be exclusively in the diaphyseal region, in the isthmic zone. In revision surgery, this type of primary stability is frequent and often imposed by a trochantero-diaphyseal flap.

NB. In an endofemoral approach, this situation is possible if the medullary canal is narrow in the isthmic zone and the cortices thick, which is rather rare in revision; the reversed situation is also possible: a wide medullary canal which imposes the selection of a large implant that is preferably anchored in the diaphyseal region.

Depending on the length of the implant, two sub-groups can be defined.

- A diaphyseal stability is called *short* when a stem of a total length of <250 mm is chosen (distal component L. 140 mm for the Revitan system) (Figs. 16.2a and 16.5). In this case, the bone/implant contact zone is approximately 3 cm.
- A diaphyseal stability is called *long* when a stem of a total length of >250 mm is chosen (distal component L. 200 mm for the Revitan system) (Fig. 16.2b). In this case, the bone/implant contact zone can be more than 4 cm.

This is usually the way to achieve primary stability with the fit and fill concept or with a self-locking stem.

NB. To define the height of the bone/implant contact zone, the length of the implant or, better, the length of the available tapered zone, if known, can serve as a reference.

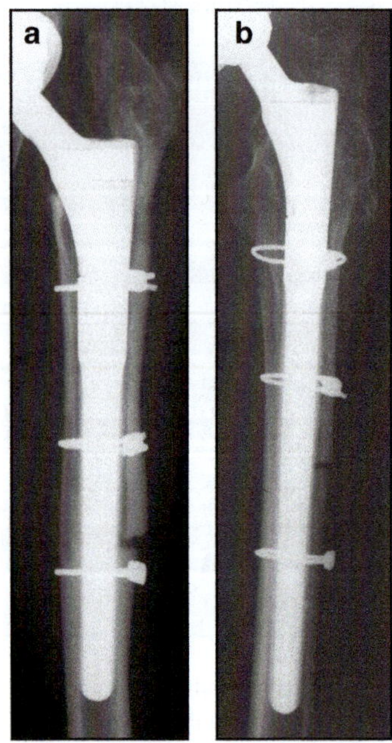

Fig. 16.2 Diaphyseal primary stability after a femoral flap: short diaphyseal stability (**a**); long diaphyseal stability (**b**)

16.1.3 Global Stability

Primary stability is achieved in the proximal and diaphyseal region of the femur.

- It is possible to achieve this fixation mode by means of an endofemoral approach (Fig. 16.3a) or after a trochanteric osteotomy if the bone stock is preserved or only slightly damaged.

   Note. Additional bone grafts or filling with other substitutes may be necessary.

- If a femoral flap has been made, we can individualize a type of ***primary diaphyseal stability globalized in the proximal femur*** if the lateral flap and the medial cortex of the femur (if necessary, after a corticotomy) are in close contact with the implant (Fig. 16.3b, c).

   Thus, different intermediate situations can be defined (globalized or not globalized diaphyseal primary stability in the proximal femur) that can be useful in identifying the factors that can have an impact on the secondary stability.

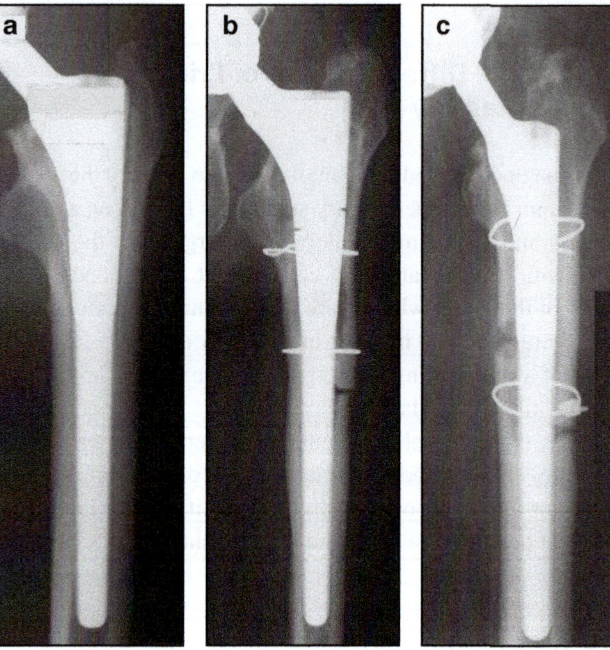

Fig. 16.3 Global primary stability: by means of an endofemoral approach (**a**), globalized diaphyseal stability after a femoral flap (**b**), globalized diaphyseal stability after a femoral flap + medial osteotomy of the cortex (**c**)

16.1.4 3-Point Stability

In this situation, there is not bone/implant contact in the form of a surface and, consequently, no true press-fit or fit and fill effect.

- When using an endofemoral approach, this situation can occur in the case of a straight stem implanted in varus in a straight femur (Fig. 16.4a) or of a straight stem in a curved femur (Fig. 16.4b).
- When making a femoral flap, this mode of primary stability remains possible. It can either be a flap that is too short to enable the reduction of a diaphyseal curvature or a long stem implanted in a femur whose diaphyseal curvature was not totally reduced (Figs. 16.4c and 16.7).

  Reminder. It is difficult to reduce a femoral curvature, even if it is not pronounced, with reamers.

  NB. There can be difficulties of interpretation if the 3-point support is located exclusively in the sagittal plane, which is often the case if a curved stem is chosen. If the femur is straight in the a/p plane, the implant may be centered but appear undersized with regard to the size of the medullary canal.

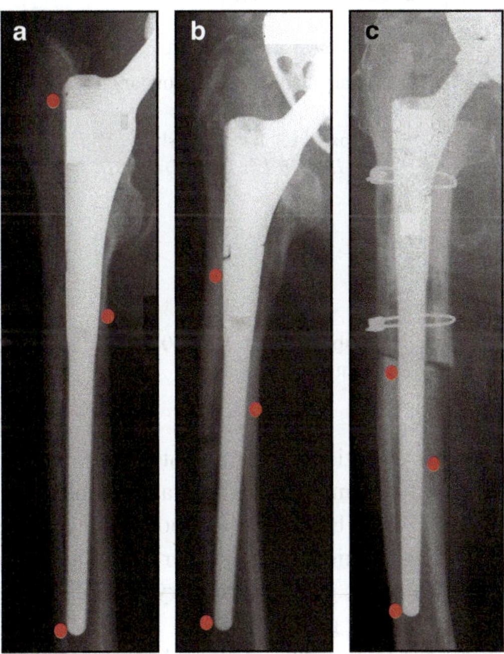

Fig. 16.4 Primary stability by means of 3-point support: (**a**) stem in varus position in a straight femur. (**b**) Straight stem in a curved femur. (**c**) Long stem in a curved femur after a femoral flap

16.2 Results

The primary stability was assessed as: proximal, 13 times (9%); global, 17 times (11%); diaphyseal short, 49 times (33%); diaphyseal long, 33 times (22%); 3-points, 38 times (25%).

16.2.1 Types of Primary Stability and Secondary Bone Stock

16.2.1.1 Results Global Series (*n 50*)
1. Qualitative Assessment

No statistically significant difference was found between secondary bone stock and the different types of primary stability, even if we group short and long diaphyseal stability (p=0.6).

Table 16.1 Primary stability and secondary bone stock

Types primary stability Secondary bone stock	Prox. (*n 13*)	Global (*n 17*)	Dia. short (*n 49*)	Dia. long (*n 33*)	3-point (*n 38*)
Very good (*n 66*)	6	6	21	14	19
Good (*n 34*)	4	6	10	5	9
Average (*n 27*)	2	3	10	5	7
Poor (*n 23*)	1	2	8	9	3

NB: Short diaphyseal stability=stem L. <250 mm and long diaphyseal stabili=stem L. >250 mm

Among the 50 patients who ultimately had a deficient secondary bone stock, the primary stability was diaphyseal in 32 patients (i.e. 64%); among the 23 cases rated as poor, 17 (i.e. 74%) had benefited from this type of primary stability; for 10 patients (i.e. 20%), primary stability was by 3-point support; global for 5 patients (i.e. 10%) and proximal for 3 patients (i.e. 6%).

Table 16.2 Evolution of the bone stock according to type of primary stability

Types primary stability **Initial bone stock**	Prox. (*n 13*)	Global (*n 17*)	Dia. short (*n 49*)	Dia. long (*n33*)	3-point (*n38*)	Types primary stability *Secondary bone stock*
Very good (*n 38*)	9–6	9–6	9–21	4–14	7–19	*Very good* (*n 66*)
Good (*n 67*)	3–4	7–6	26–10	15–5	16–9	*Good* (*n 34*)
Average (*n 38*)	1–2	1–3	13–10	10–5	13–7	*Average* (*n 27*)
Poor (*n 7*)	0–1	0–2	1–8	4–9	2–3	*Poor* (*n 23*)

NB: Short diaphyseal stability=stem L.<250 mm and long diaphyseal stability=stem L.>250 mm

A significant correlation between initial and secondary bone stock was only observed in cases with so-called global primary stability (p=0.04). The same correlation could not be found in the other types of primary stability (proximal: p=0.3; diaphyseal: p=0.5; 3-point: p=0.2).

2. Numerical Assessment (Results and Evolution)

Table 16.3 Initial bone stock progresses little (14.5/20 vs 14.7/20 at the last follow-up)

Types primary stability / Bone stock	Prox. (*n 13*)	Global (*n 17*)	Dia. short (*n 49*)	Dia. long (*n 33*)	3-point (*n 38*)	Total (*n 150*)
Initial bone stock	16.9	17	14.4	13.2	13.7	**14.5**
Secondary bone stock	15.5	15.1	14.8	13	15.3	**14.7**
Difference	−1.4	−1.9	+0.4	−0.2	+1.6	**+0.2**

NB: Short diaphyseal stability = stem L. < 250 mm and long diaphyseal stability = stem L. > 250 mm

The evolution of bone stock varies significantly between one type of primary stability and another (p < 0.0001).

NB. A numerical evaluation is finer and more precise than recoding by class, and less information is lost.

16.2.1.2 Deficient Bone Stock (*n 50*) According to Length of Implant and Type of Primary Stability

In the sub-group average/poor secondary bone stock (*n* = 50), the statistical study does not indicate a significant difference between the deficiency of secondary bone stock and the length of the implant (<200 mm vs >200 mm) (p = 0.4), nor between the type of primary stability (diaphyseal/3-point vs global/proximal) and the length of the implant (p = 0.9); on the other hand, in a statistical study between diaphyseal stability versus global/proximal/3-point and the length of the implant, a borderline significant difference is found (p = 0.07).

Table 16.4 Bone stock deficient (*n 50*) according to length of implant and primary stability

Implant length (*in mm*)		
Types primary stability	L. < 200	L. > 200
Diaphyseal (*n 32*)	9	23
3-points (*n 10*)	0	10
Global (*n 5*)	1	4
Proximal (*n 3*)	0	3

In the sub-group of 50 patients with deficient secondary bone stock, if a femoral stem of L. >200 mm was chosen and a diaphyseal primary stability was achieved, 72% of the patients (i.e. 23 vs 32 patients) have deficient secondary bone stock.

Conversely, selecting a stem of L. <200 mm seems to favor the preservation of bone stock or to limit its degradation, except when the primary stability is diaphyseal.

Moreover, a globalized diaphyseal primary stability by seeking additional proximal stability of the implant does not seem to be a decisive factor to preserve or regenerate bone stock (Fig. 16.5). Of the 32 cases with diaphyseal primary stability and deficient secondary bone stock, 19 had enjoyed proximal stability and 13 cases had not had any proximal stability (Fig. 16.6).

In Summary

1. On average, an increase of bone stock is limited: difference of +0.2 point.
2. Proximal or global fixation does not prevent the degradation of bone stock, however, bone stock degrades often less.
3. Within the group of diaphyseal primary stability, the strongest progression can be observed in the cases rated as poor; they increase from 5 to 17 cases.
4. Implantation of a long stem, within the framework of a diaphyseal primary stability, seems to be less beneficial for the bone stock.
5. 3-point stability is not an obstacle to the regeneration of bone stock (Fig. 16.7).

16.2.2 Types of Primary Stability and Secondary Stability

16.2.2.1 Results Global Series (*n 150*)
1. Quantitative Assessment

Patients who ultimately had a lack of secondary stability (weighted score) enjoyed significantly more often diaphyseal primary stability (p = 0.05).

Table 16.5 Types primary stability and secondary stability

Types primary stability / Secondary stability	Prox. (*n 13*)	Global (*n 17*)	Dia. short (*n 49*)	Dia. long (*n 33*)	3-point (*n 38*)
Very good (*n 83*)	11	12	27	13	20
Good (*n 41*)	1	5	10	12	13
Average (*n 19*)	1	/	9	6	3
Poor (*n 7*)	/	/	3	2	2

NB: Short diaphyseal stability = stem L. <250 mm and long diaphyseal stability = stem L. >250 mm

Among the 26 patients who ultimately had deficient secondary stability, primary stability was : diaphyseal in 20 patients (i.e. 77%); by 3-point support in 5 patients (i.e. 19%); in 1 single patient (4%), primary stability was proximal, and when it was global, secondary stability was always rated as very good or good.

With regard to the 37 patients who had deficient secondary osseointegration in the proximal portion of the implant and which were rated as « good » after weighting (and who, thus, are not part of this group of 26 patients rated as average/poor), 31 patients (i.e. 84%) had diaphyseal or 3-point primary stability ; only 6 patients (i.e. 16%) belong to the group of proximal or global primary stability.

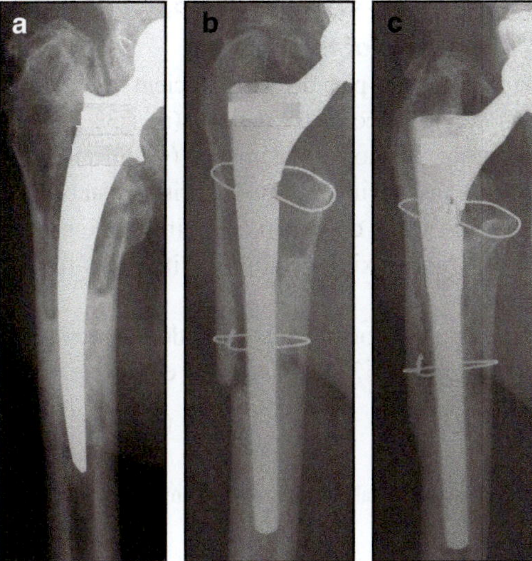

Fig. 16.5 A 81-year-old female patient, loosening accompanied by a destruction of the bone stock of the proximal femur , IC very good 0.60 (**a**). Revision by transfemoral approach, diaphyseal primary stability with a short stem, no additional bone graft and gap + of the femoral flap (**b**). At the 5-year follow-up, good regeneration of the bone stock. Score for secondary bone stock: good 16/20. No lucent lines. Secondary stability 20/20 (**c**). **G**lobal **R**adiographic **S**core: good 18/20. **NB**. It may be assumed that the regeneration of bone stock was favored by a favorable bone condition and by non-aggressive surgery with respect to vascular integrity (no periosteal stripping) and implantation of a short stem

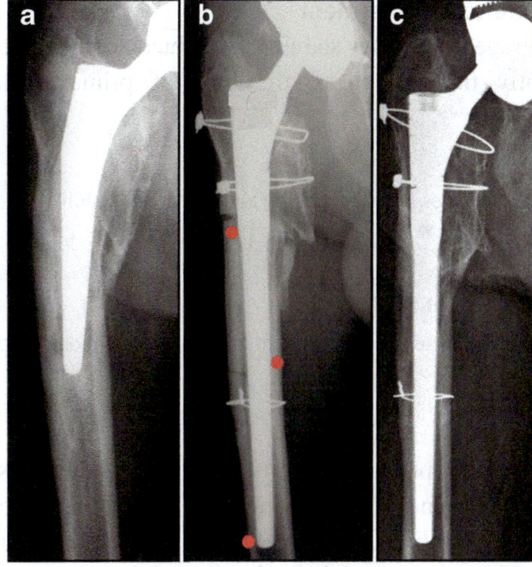

Fig. 16.7 A 65-year-old male patient, loosening with pronounced varus curvature of the proximal femur following fracture (**a**). Revision by a trochanteric osteotomy enlarged and femoral window. Primary stability by means of three-point support with a long stem, no additional bone grafting, osteotomy of the medial cortex (**b**). At the 13-year follow-up, perfect osseointegration of the entire implant, secondary global stability 2 +, very good: 20/20. Secondary bone stock: 18/20, slight decrease of the bone density in zone 6 (**c**). **G**lobal **R**adiographic **S**core: very good 20/20. **NB**. In this case, a trochantero-diaphyseal flap of approximately 16 cm would have been preferable, would have facilitated implantation of a shorter stem and avoided three-point fixation

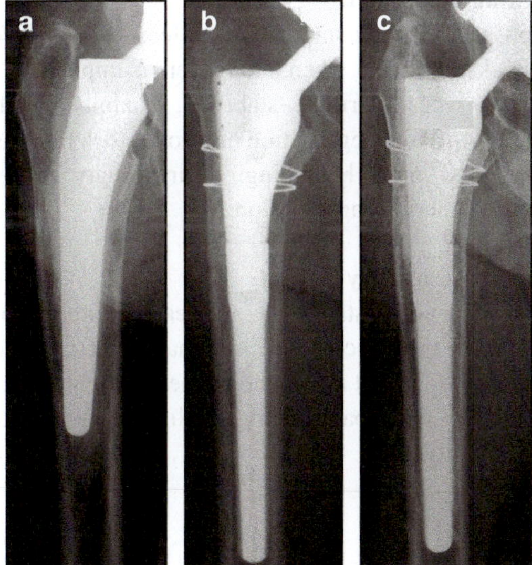

Fig. 16.6 A 71-year-old female patient, no significant defects of the bone stock (some granulomas in the medial cortex), straight femur but IC poor 0. 33 (**a**). Endofemoral approach, proximal primary stability with insertion of endomedullary bone grafts and cerclage of the proximal femur (**b**). At the 6-year follow-up, stable prosthesis, no lucent lines. Score for secondary stability 20/20. Bone stock preserved, slight decrease of the bone density in zone 6. Score 18/20 (**c**). **G**lobal **R**adiographic **S**core: very good 20/20

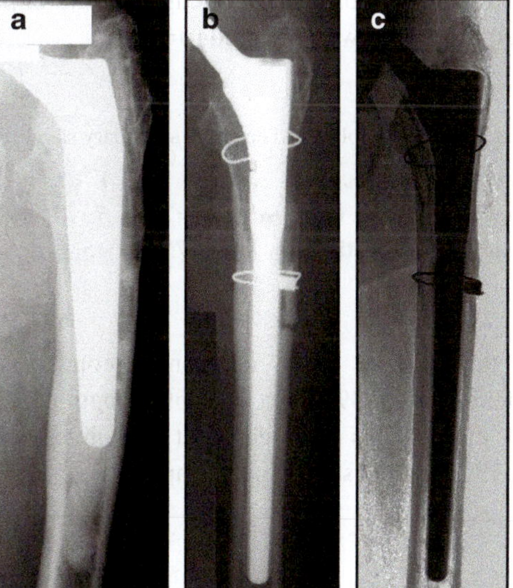

Fig. 16.8 A 71-year-old female patient, loosening, varus curvature of the femur, destruction of the lateral cortex, cement plug (**a**). Revision by transfemoral approach, primary stability by means of diaphyseal press-fit with a long stem (265 mm), no additional bone grafting nor proximal stabilization (no osteotomy of the medial cortex) (**b**). At the 7-year follow-up, distinct radiolucent line >50% in the proximal femur, distal secondary stability +, average: 11/20. Average secondary bone stock: 12/20, no regeneration in zone 1, decrease of the bone density in zones 2 and 3 (**c**). **G**lobal **R**adiographic **S**core: poor 10/20. **NB**. In this situation, it would have been preferable to implant a short stem and to perform an osteotomy of the medial cortex as well as insert additional bone grafts or other bone substitutes

2. Numerical Assessment

On average, secondary stability (weighted score) varies significantly in function of the type of primary stability ($p < 0.0001$).

Table 16.6 Types primary stability and secondary stability

Types primary stability	Prox. (*n 13*)	Global (*n 17*)	Dia. short (*n 49*)	Dia. long (*n33*)	3-point (*n38*)
Secondary stability	**18.5**	**18**	**16.3**	**15.3**	**16.4**

NB: Short diaphyseal stability = stem L. <250 mm and long diaphyseal stability = stem L. >250 mm

Diaphyseal primary stability (especially when it is considered long) and 3-point fixation are the least favorable for secondary stability. On the other hand, proximal primary stability (Fig. 16.6) or global primary stability foster perfect secondary stability of the implant.

16.2.2.2 Deficient Stability and Length of Implant < or > 200 mm

- In the sub-group of patients with deficient secondary stability $n = 26$ (weighted score), no significant correlation between the length of the implant and secondary stability was found ($p = 0.4$).
- The same can be said for the sub-group of patients with deficient osseointegration $n = 73$ (raw score): no significant correlation between the length of the implant and osseointegration was observed ($p = 0.9$).

Table 16.7 Length implant and deficient secondary stability

Length of implant (*in mm*)	L. < 200	L. > 200
Deficient second. stab. (*weighted sc.*) $n = 26$	7	19
Deficient osseointegration (*raw sc.*) $n = 73$	15	58

Of the patients with deficient secondary stability (weighted score), 73% had a stem of a length of >200 mm, and of the patients with deficient osseointegration (raw score), 79% had the same type of implant.

16.2.2.3 Deficient Stability and Proximal Stability of the Implant

- In the sub-group of patients with deficient secondary stability $n = 26$ (weighted score), 19 patients (i.e. 73%) did not have proximal stabilization of the implant (significant $p < 0.0001$).

  Nb. 14 cases with diaphyseal primary stability have to be added to the 5 cases with 3-point fixation, where, by definition, no proximal stability with press-fit effect can be achieved.
- In the sub-group of patients with deficient osseointegration (raw score $n = 73$), this trend is confirmed (significant $p < 0.0001$).

Table 16.8 Proximal stabilization of implant and deficient secondary stability

Proximal stabilization	Yes	No
Deficient second. stab. (*weighted sc.*) $n = 26$	7 (27%)	19 (73%)
Deficient osseointegration (*raw sc.*) $n = 73$	27 (37%)	46 (63%)

- When there is no proximal stabilization, choosing a long stem (L. >250 mm) has a negative impact: of the 13 patients who had received such an implant, 12 ultimately had deficient osseointegration (significant $p = 0.002$) (Fig. 16.8).

In Summary

Regarding bone stock

A diaphyseal primary stability is the least favorable for the bone stock, especially when a long stem is implanted.

The two types of primary stability , proximal and global , do not help to avoid degradation of a bone stock rated as very good or good in the beginning. Their primary virtue is to avoid further serious aggravation.

Regarding secondary stability

Diaphyseal primary stability is the least favorable for secondary stability, especially if proximal stabilization of the implant is not assured at the end of the intervention. In contrast, proximal or global primary stability is beneficial to secondary stability.

Degree of Osteoporosis and Its Impact on the Radiographic Results (Bone Stock and Secondary Stability)

A preoperative assessment of the degree of osteoporosis (or bone condition) is crucial when an uncemented stem is chosen, especially in revision surgery.

In addition to increasing the difficulties encountered in revision surgery (via falsa, fracture, incomplete cement excision), osteoporosis can induce bone changes and, eventually, be at the origin of severe alterations of the bone stock.

Reminder. The assessment of the degree of osteoporosis is described in part 2: on an a/p radiograph, the geometry of the medullary canal is evaluated and the thickness of the cortices is also measured by means of a Cortical Index (CI). In the end, a classification into four stages is done.

17.1 Results

The degree of osteoporosis was rated: St.1-Very good (CI =/>0.55) 30 times (20%); St.2-Good (CI 0.45 to 0.54) 46 times (31%); St.3-Average (CI 0.35 to 0.44) 56 times (37%); St.4-Poor (CI =/<0.34) 18 times (12%).

17.1.1 Osteoporosis and Secondary Bone Stock

17.1.1.1 Results Global Series (*n* 150)
Qualitative Assessment

A significant correlation was found between the degree of osteoporosis and secondary bone stock (p<0.0001).

Table 17.1 Osteoporosis and secondary bone stock

Osteoporosis stage Secondary bone stock	St.1- VG (*n 30*)	St.2- G (*n 46*)	St.3- Av (*n 56*)	St.4- P (*n 18*)
Very good (*n 66*)	24	21	19	2
Good (*n 34*)	5	16	10	3
Average (*n 27*)	1	8	16	2
Poor (*n 23*)	/	1	11	11

In the presence of osteoporosis, the evolution of bone stock is not favorable: 40 of the 50 patients (i.e. 80%) who had a deficient bone stock at the last follow-up, had initially been diagnosed with an established osteoporosis stage 3 and 4.

Referring to the 4 stages of osteoporosis: 72% of the cases stage 4 had deficient secondary bone stock; this percentage is 48% for an osteoporosis stage 3; 19% for an osteoporosis stage 2 and 3% for an osteoporosis stage 1.

Numerical Assessment
The average progression of the bone stock varies significantly depending on the stage of osteoporosis (p<0.0001).

Table 17.2 Osteoporosis and secondary bone stock

Value bone stock Osteoporosis stage	Initial	Secondary	Difference
St.1- Very good (*n 30*)	16.2	18.3	**+2.1**
St.2- Good (*n 46*)	15	15.9	**+0.9**
St.3- Average (*n 56*)	13.6	13.5	**−0.1**
St.4- Poor (*n 18*)	13.3	8.6	**−4.7**

It is important to note an increase of +2.1 points in the absence of osteoporosis (16.2 vs 18.3 points) and a reduction of −4.7 points in the presence of osteoporosis stage 4 (13.3 vs 8.6 points).

Note. These numbers underline again the benefits of a numerical evaluation that shows more significant differences which are sometimes difficult to detect in a qualitative assessment.

17.1.1.2 Secondary Bone Stock in Relation to Osteoporosis Stage
Osteoporosis Stage 1 (*n* 30)

In this sub-group of patients, no significant correlation between initial and secondary bone stock has been observed (p=0.2).

Table 17.3 Secondary bone stock and osteoporosis stage 1

	Secondary bone stock					
	Average/poor		VG/good		Total	
Initial bone stock	Nb	%	Nb	%	Nb	%
Average/poor	/	/	4	100.0	4	13.3
Very good/good	1	3.8	25	96.2	26	86.7
Total	1	3.3	29	96.7	30	100.0

P. Le Béguec et al., *Uncemented Femoral Stems for Revision Surgery*,
DOI 10.1007/978-3-319-03614-4_17, © Springer International Publishing Switzerland 2015

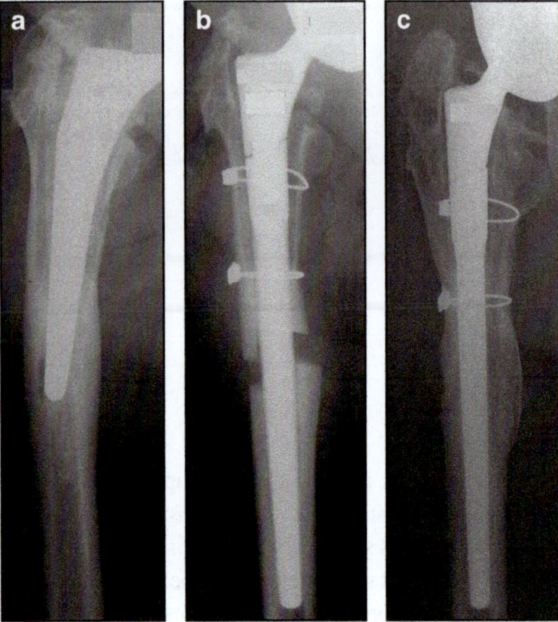

Fig. 17.1 A 76-year-old female patient, loosening with varus curvature of the femur, no osteoporosis: CI rated as good at 0.50 (**a**). Revision by trochantero-diaphyseal flap and osteotomy of the medial cortex, diaphyseal primary stability with a long stem. Significant gap at the level of the osteotomy and thinned cortex + in zone 6; initial bone stock average 12/20 (**b**). At the 5-year follow-up, deficient proximal osseointegration, proximal secondary stability −, good: 14/20. Filling of the bone defects and regeneration of the medial cortex, secondary bone stock: 20/20 (**c**). Global Radiographic Score: good 18/20

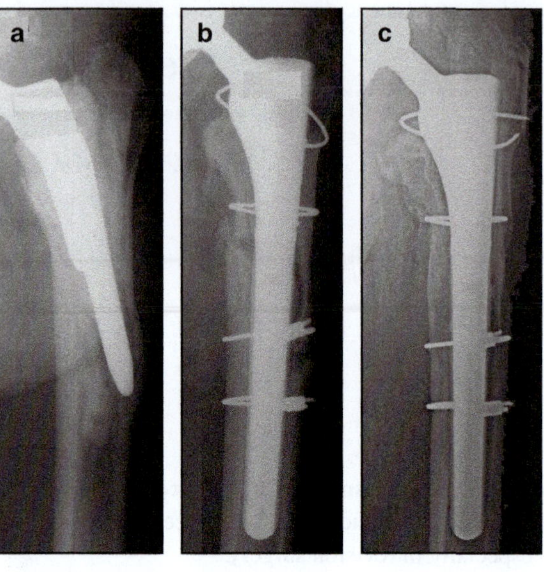

Fig. 17.3 A 71-year-old female patient, iterative loosening with severely impaired bone stock, curved femur, osteoporosis: CI rated stage 4, poor at 0.30 (**a**). Revision by trochantero-diaphyseal flap, diaphyseal primary stability with a long stem of large diameter (20 mm), cortical defect in zone 2 (**b**). At the 8-year follow-up, no regeneration in zone 2 and marked decrease of the bone density of the entire femur with cortical thinning in zones 3 and 5; secondary bone stock poor: 0/20. Distal secondary stability +, average: 11/20 (**c**). Global Radiographic Score: poor 7/20. NB: the distal bone plug at 8 years, probably due to significant stiffening of the bone/implant couple and a sudden rupture of the cortical bone elasticity

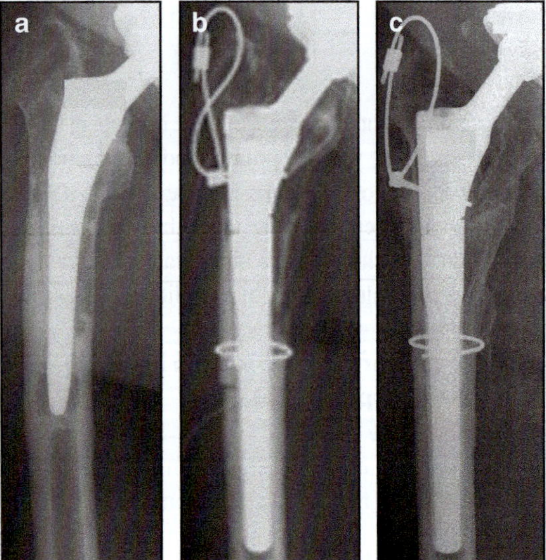

Fig. 17.2 A 77-year-old female patient, loosening with granulomas ++, varus curvature of the femur, no osteoporosis: CI rated as good at 0.51 (**a**). Revision by trochantero-diaphyseal flap, osteotomy and fracture of the medial cortex, diaphyseal primary stability with a short stem. Impairment of greater trochanter and zone 6, fracture of the medial cortex with gap +; initial bone stock average 10/20 (**b**). At the 5-year follow-up, perfect osseointegration, global secondary stability 2+, very good: 20/20. Filling of the bone defects and regeneration of the medial cortex, persistent deficit ± at the level of the greater trochanter. Secondary bone stock: 18/20 (**c**). Global Radiographic Score: very good 20/20

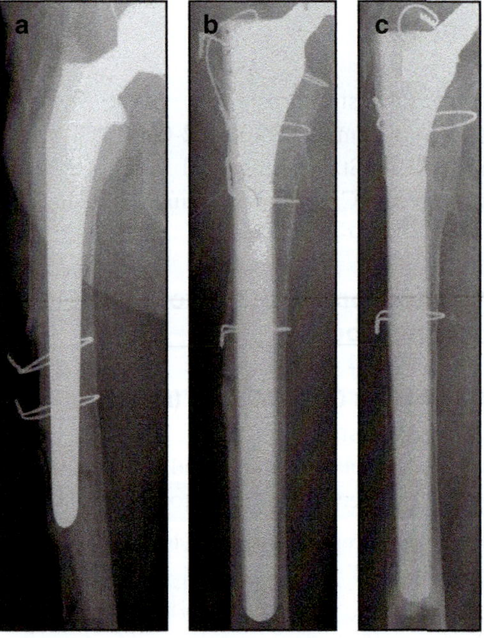

Fig. 17.4 A 70-year-old male patient, iterative loosening, defect of the lateral cortex in zone 2, curved femur, osteoporosis ± stage 3 average, CI 0.42 (**a**). Revision by trochantero-diaphyseal flap and osteotomy of the medial cortex, diaphyseal primary stability with a short stem (**b**). At the 9-year follow-up, decrease ± of the bone density in zones 2, 3, 5 and 6 without decrease of cortical thickness. Secondary bone stock average: 12/20 (**c**). Global secondary stability +/−, good: 14/20 (fibrous fixation?). Global Radiographic Score: average 13/20. **NB**. In this case (iterative loosening) it may be assumed that additional bone grafting or another substitute would have been beneficial

In the absence of osteoporosis, an initial bone stock rated as average/poor can become very good/good at a later stage (Figs. 17.1 and 17.2), and a bone stock initially rated as very good/good may deteriorate.

Osteoporosis Stage 4 (*n* 18)

In this sub-group of patients, a significant correlation between initial and secondary bone stock was found (p=0.03).

Table 17.4 Secondary bone stock and osteoporosis stage 4

	Secondary bone stock					
	Average/poor		VG/good		Total	
Initial bone stock	Nb	%	Nb	%	Nb	%
Average/poor	6	85.7	1	14,3	7	38.9
Very good/good	7	63.6	4	36.4	11	61.1
Total	13	72.2	5	27.8	18	100.0

The more the initial bone stock is rated as very good/good in the presence of osteoporosis, the more it will be very good/good in a second phase, and an initially poor bone stock shows a tendency to remain poor (Fig. 17.3).

In this situation, it is especially necessary to avoid a worsening of the bone stock!

17.1.2 Osteoporosis and Secondary Stability

Results Global Series (*n* 150)
Qualitative Assessment

No significant correlation between the degree of osteoporosis and secondary stability (weighted score) could be found (p=0.3).

Osteoporosis stage	St.1- VG	St.2- G	St.3- Av	St.4- P
Secondary stability	(*n 30*)	(*n 46*)	(*n 56*)	(*n 18*)
Very good (*n 83*)	20	24	28	11
Good (*n 41*)	5	16	15	5
Average (*n 19*)	3	6	8	2
Poor (*n 7*)	2	/	5	/

Of the 26 patients who ultimately had deficient secondary stability, 13 (i.e. 50%) have an osteoporosis stage 3, and only 2 patients who had been rated average (8%) belong to the group with osteoporosis stage 4.

Numerical Assessment

The results for secondary stability (weighted score) obtained in function of the degree of osteoporosis show a signification difference depending on the stage of osteoporosis (p<0.0001).

Table 17.5 Osteoporosis and secondary stability

	St.1- VG	St.2- G	St.3- Av	St.4- Mv
Osteoporosis stage	(*n 30*)	(*n 46*)	(*n 56*)	(*n 18*)
Secondary stability	17	16.6	**15.9**	17.6

Patients classified as osteoporosis stage 3 (average) had the weakest arithmetic mean (Fig. 17.4); in contrast, osteoporosis stage 4 (poor) has no negative impact on osseointegration.

These results confirm those obtained in qualitative version.

17.1.3 Osteoporosis Stage 3–4 (*n* 74)

Table 17.6 Osteoporosis stage 3–4 (*n* 74): secondary bone stock and secondary stability according to the type of primary stability

Types primary stability	Prox. (*n 6*)	Global (*n 6*)	Dia. short (*n 21*)	Dia. long (*n 22*)	3-point (*n 19*)
Secondary bone stock					
Very good (*n 21*)	4	1	4	7	5
Good (*n 13*)	/	1	4	3	5
Average (*n 18*)	1	2	6	3	6
Poor (*n 22*)	1	2	7	9	3
Secondary stability (*weighted score*)					
Very good (*39*)	6	5	14	6	8
Good (*n 20*)	/	1	3	9	7
Average (*n 10*)	/	/	2	5	3
Poor (*n 5*)	/	/	2	2	1

NB: Short diaphyseal stability=stem L.<250 mm and long diaphyseal stability=stem L.>250 mm

17.1.3.1 Secondary Bone Stock

- In this sub-group, the correlation between secondary bone stock and degree of osteoporosis remains significant (p<0.0001) (see paragraph 1).

  In the presence of osteoporosis, the percentage of the cases rated as average/poor increases (54% vs 33% if the reference is the entire cohort of 150 patients).

Table 17.7 Osteoporosis stage 3–4: secondary bone stock according to primary stability

	Type of primary stability					
	Diaphyseal		Other		Total	
Second. bone stock	Nb	%	Nb	%	Nb	%
Average/poor	25	62.5	15	37,5	26	38.9
Very good/good	18	52.9	16	47.1	124	61.1
Total	43	58.1	31	41.9	150	100.0

- In contrast, no significant correlation was found between secondary bone stock (very good/good versus average/poor) and the type or primary stability (diaphyseal versus other) (p = 0.4). However, it must be noted that among the 43 patients who had experienced diaphyseal primary stability, 25 (i.e. 62.5%) ultimately had deficient secondary bone stock; in 11 cases, this was due to a decrease in bone density in combination with decreased cortical thickness.

17.1.3.2 Secondary Stability

The presence of osteoporosis does not significantly increase the percentage of deficient secondary stability (20% versus 17% for the entire cohort of 150 patients), and no significant correlation could be found between the type of primary stability (diaphyseal versus other) and secondary stability (very good/good versus average/poor) (p = 0.2).

In Summary

Regarding bone stock

The absence of osteoporosis is beneficial for the preservation and/or regeneration of bone stock. In contrast, the presence of osteoporosis stage 4 is very unfavorable, and in this situation, the press-fit concept can be contraindicated if proximal primary stability cannot be achieved.

Regarding secondary stability

The presence of osteoporosis stage 4 does not have a negative impact on secondary stability, however, it must be underlined that this is at the expense of the bone stock - through a decrease of the bone density and often the thickness of the cortices- if the primary stability is in the diaphyseal region.

In the presence of osteoporosis stage 3, it is important to remain vigilant and, whenever possible, to give priority to a proximal fixation of the implant. If necessary, additional bone grafts, possibly associated with osseoinductive or osseoconductive factors.

Deficient Initial Bone Stock and its Impact on the Radiographic Results (Bone Stock and Secondary Stability)

In revision surgery, the initial bone stock is a factor that can have an impact on secondary bone stock and secondary stability. It also serves as a reference in the evaluation of the bone prior to surgery.

Reminder: The method to evaluate initial and secondary bone stock is described in the first part. For every Gruen zone, the following is evaluated: thickness of the cortices,

Results

The initial bone stock was rated as: very good, 38 times (25%); good, 67 times (45%); average, 38 times (25%), and poor, 7 times (5%).

18.1 Value of Initial and Secondary Bone Stock

18.1.1 Results Global Series (*n* 150)

Qualitative Assessment

No significant correlation was found between initial and secondary bone stock (p=0.5).

Table 18.1 Initial bone stock and secondary bone stock

Initial bone stock Secondary bone stock	Very good (*n 38*)	Good (*n 67*)	Average (*n 38*)	Poor (*n 7*)
Very good (*n 66*)	23	33	9	1
Good (*n 34*)	10	10	13	1
Average (*n 27*)	3	16	7	1
Poor (*n 23*)	2	8	9	4

In 47% of the cases (i.e. 21 patients), an initial bone stock rated as average and poor (45 patients) did not show improvement, and the initial bone stock rated as very good/good (105 patients) deteriorated in 28% cases (i.e. 29 patients). Ultimately, an increase of the cases rated as average/poor is observed (50 versus 45), with an increase, particularly, of the cases rated as poor, which were 7 in the beginning and 23 at the last follow-up.

Numerical Assessment

A statistically significant difference between initial and secondary bone stock can be found (p<0.0001).

Table 18.2 Evolution of bone stock (*numerical values*)

Bone stock	Initial	Second	Difference
Very good (*n 38*)	18.5	16.7	−1.8
Good (*n 67*)	14.9	15	+0.1
Average (*n 38*)	11.1	13	+1.9
Poor (*n 7*)	7	8.5	+1.5

A bone stock rated as very good in the beginning can deteriorate in proportions that remain, however, moderate, and initially impaired bone stock can regenerate in a way that is not always very spectacular.

18.1.2 Deficient Initial Bone Stock (*n* 45): Secondary Bone Stock Depending on the Stage of Osteoporosis

Qualitative Assessment

In the sub-group of 45 patients with deficient initial bone stock, there is a significant correlation between secondary bone stock and the stage of osteoporosis (p=0.007).

Table 18.3 Deficient initial bone stock (*n* 45): osteoporosis and secondary bone stock

Stages osteoporosis Secondary bone stock	St.1: VG (*n 4*)	St.2: G (*n 9*)	St.3: Av (*n 25*)	St.4: P (*n 7*)
Very good (*n=10*)	1	3	6	/
Good (*n=14*)	3	4	6	1
Average (*n=8*)	/	1	7	/
Poor (*n=13*)	/	1	6	6

P. Le Béguec et al., *Uncemented Femoral Stems for Revision Surgery*,
DOI 10.1007/978-3-319-03614-4_18, © Springer International Publishing Switzerland 2015

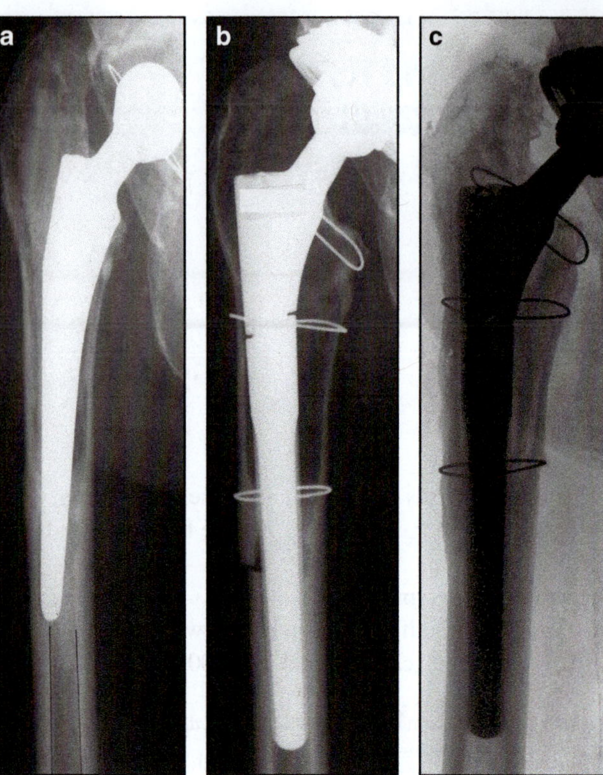

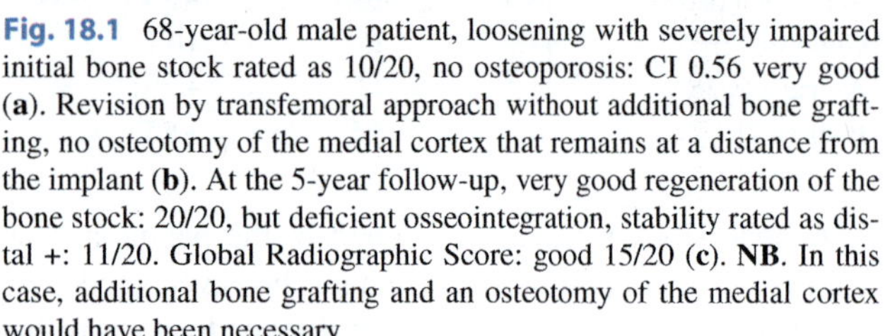

Fig. 18.1 68-year-old male patient, loosening with severely impaired initial bone stock rated as 10/20, no osteoporosis: CI 0.56 very good (**a**). Revision by transfemoral approach without additional bone grafting, no osteotomy of the medial cortex that remains at a distance from the implant (**b**). At the 5-year follow-up, very good regeneration of the bone stock: 20/20, but deficient osseointegration, stability rated as distal +: 11/20. Global Radiographic Score: good 15/20 (**c**). **NB**. In this case, additional bone grafting and an osteotomy of the medial cortex would have been necessary

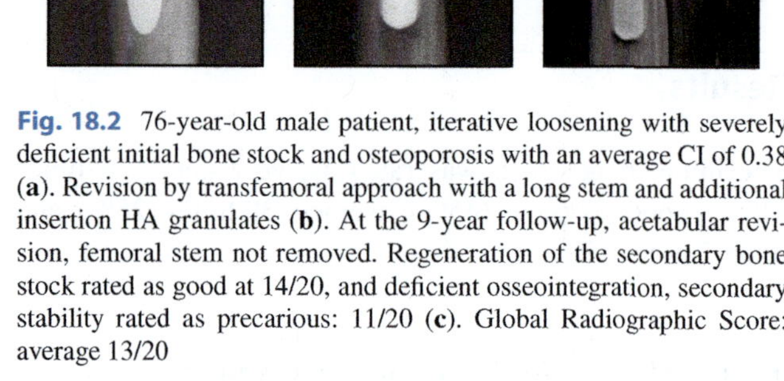

Fig. 18.2 76-year-old male patient, iterative loosening with severely deficient initial bone stock and osteoporosis with an average CI of 0.38 (**a**). Revision by transfemoral approach with a long stem and additional insertion HA granulates (**b**). At the 9-year follow-up, acetabular revision, femoral stem not removed. Regeneration of the secondary bone stock rated as good at 14/20, and deficient osseointegration, secondary stability rated as precarious: 11/20 (**c**). Global Radiographic Score: average 13/20

In the absence of osteoporosis, regeneration of the initial bone stock, with ultimately a bone stock rated as very good or good, has been possible for 11 of the 13 patients (i.e. 85%) that had a deficient bone stock in the beginning (Fig. 18.1).

In the presence of osteoporosis, regeneration of the initial bone stock seems more random as 19 of the 32 patients (i.e. 60%) who were evaluated as average/poor in the beginning kept the same rating. It must be underlined, however, that bone regeneration remains possible in 40% of the patients (13 versus 32). The unfavorable impact of an osteoporosis (stage 3–4) does not significantly impede the regeneration of the bone stock that was impaired in the beginning, especially if certain surgical precautions are taken (Fig. 18.2).

Numerical Assessment

In the sub-group of 45 patients with deficient initial bone stock, the value of secondary bone stock, on average numerical, varies significantly, depending on the presence or not of osteoporosis ($p = 0.03$).

Table 18.4 Deficient initial bone stock: osteoporosis and secondary bone stock (*numerical values*)

Deficient initial bone stock	No osteoporosis (*n 13*)	Osteoporosis (*n 32*)
Secondary bone stock	15.2	11.1

18.1.3 Deficient Initial Bone Stock (*n* 45): Secondary Bone Stock According to Type of Primary Stability

In the sub-group of 45 patients with deficient initial bone stock, the distribution between secondary bone stock and the different types of primary stability does not reveal a significant difference (p=0.7). It must, however, be underlined that, of the 13 patients evaluated as "poor secondary bone stock", 10 patients (i.e. 77%) had diaphyseal primary stability (p=0.3).

Table 18.5 Deficient initial bone stock (*n* 45): secondary bone stock according primary stability

Primary stability	Prox.	Global	Dia. short	Dia. long	3-point
Secondary bone stock	(*n 1*)	(*n 1*)	(*n 14*)	(*n 14*)	(*n 15*)
Very good (*n 10*)	/	/	4	4	2
Good (*n 14*)	1	/	3	3	7
Average (*n 8*)	/	/	3	1	4
Poor (*n 13*)	/	1	4	6	2

Nb. The small number of cases with proximal and global primary stability is logical considering the patient population of this study (with deficient initial bone stock)

18.2 Value of Initial Bone Stock and Secondary Stability

18.2.1 Results Global Series (*n* 150)

Qualitative Assessment
A significant correlation can be found between initial bone stock and secondary stability (weighted score) (p=0.04).

Table 18.6 Initial bone stock and secondary stability

Initial bone stock	Very good	Good	Average	Poor
Secondary stability	(*n 38*)	(*n 67*)	(*n 38*)	(*n 7*)
Very good (*n 83*)	28	36	17	2
Good (*n 41*)	6	22	11	2
Average (*n 19*)	2	7	8	2
Poor (*n 7*)	2	2	2	1

Among the 26 patients who ultimately had a deficient secondary stability, an even distribution between patients who had a deficient bone stock in the beginning, and those whose initial bone stock had been preserved, must be noted.

Numerical Assessment
The value of secondary stability (weighted score) varies significantly depending on the initial bone stock (p <0.0001).

Table 18.7 Initial bone stock and secondary stability (*numerical values*)

Initial bone stock	Very good (*n 38*)	Good (*n 67*)	Average (*n 38*)	Poor (*n 7*)
Secondary stability	17.7	16.6	15.6	14

18.2.2 Deficient Initial Bone Stock (*n* 45): Secondary Stability Depending on the Stage of Osteoporosis

- In the sub-group of 45 patients who had a deficient initial bone stock, the distribution between secondary stability (weighted score) and the degree of osteoporosis does not reveal any significant difference (p=0.9).

Table 18.8 Deficient initial bone stock (*n* 45): secondary stability according to osteoporosis

Osteoporosis stages	St.1: VG	St.2: G	St.3: Av	St.4: P
Secondary stability	(*n 4*)	(*n 9*)	(*n 25*)	(*n 7*)
Very good (*n=19*)	2	3	11	3
Good (*n=13*)	1	3	7	2
Average (*n=10*)	1	3	4	2
Poor (*n=3*)	/	/	3	/

- The results with the numerical values confirm the non-significant role of the presence of osteoporosis for secondary stability (weighted score) p=0.9.

Table 18.9 Deficient initial bone stock (*n* 45): secondary stability according to osteoporosis (*numerical values*)

Deficient initial bone stock	No osteoporosis (*n 13*)	Osteoporosis (*n 32*)
Secondary stability	15.3	15.4

18.2.3 Deficient Initial Bone Stock (*n* 45): Secondary Stability Depending on the Type of Primary Stability

- In the sub-group of 45 patients with deficient initial bone stock, the distribution of secondary stability (weighted score) and the different types of primary stability (diaphyseal versus other) does not reveal any significant differences (p=0.7).

Table 18.10 Deficient initial bone stock (*n* 45): secondary stability according primary stability

Primary stability Secondary stability	Prox. (*n 1*)	Global (*n 1*)	Dia. short (*n 14*)	Dia. long (*n 14*)	3-point (*n 15*)
Very good (*n 19*)	/	/	9	4	6
Good (*n 13*)	/	1	2	4	6
Average (*n 10*)	1	/	3	4	2
Poor (*n 3*)	/	/	/	2	1

Short diaphyseal stability = stem L. <250 mm and long diaphyseal stability = stem L. >250 mm

Of the 13 patients who ultimately had deficient secondary stability (weighted score), it must be noted that 9 patients (i.e. 69%) had diaphyseal primary stability in the beginning.

- In this same sub-group, the results in numerical values (diayphseal stability versus other) confirm the non-significant role of the type of primary stability (p=0.8).

Table 18.11 Deficient initial bone stock (*n* 45): primary stability and secondary stability (*numerical values*)

Deficient initial bone stock	Diaphyseal stability (*n 28*)	Other (*n 17*)
Secondary stability	15.6	15.1

18.3 Deficient Initial Bone Stock + Osteoporosis (*n* 32): Secondary Bone Stock and Stability Depending on the Primary Stability

18.3.1 Secondary Bone Stock

The association of deficient initial bone stock and osteoporosis significantly increases the percentage of cases rated as secondary bone stock average/poor: 59% versus 13% in the absence of osteoporosis and impaired initial bone stock (p=0.0004).

18.3.2 Secondary Stability

The association of deficient initial bone stock and osteoporosis changes the percentage of cases evaluated as having an average/poor secondary stability only little, i.e. 28% versus 31% in the absence of osteoporosis, and the distribution of

Table 18.12 Deficient initial bone stock and osteoporosis (*n* 32): secondary bone stock and secondary stability according to primary stability

Deficient initial bone stock + osteoporosis	Prox. (*n 0*)	Global (*n 1*)	D. short (*n 8*)	D. long (*n 12*)	3-point (*n 11*)
Secondary bone stock					
Very good (*n 6*)	/	/	2	3	1
Good (*n 7*)	/	/	1	2	4
Average (*n 7*)	/	/	2	1	4
Poor (*n 12*)	/	1	3	6	2
Secondary stability (*weighted score*)					
Very good (*n 14*)	/	/	6	4	4
Good (*n 9*)	/	1	1	3	4
Average (*n 6*)	/	/	1	3	2
Poor (*n 3*)	/	/	/	2	1

Short diaphyseal stability = stem L. <250 mm and long diaphyseal stability = stem L. >250 mm

secondary stability (weighted score) and the different types of primary stability (diaphyseal and other) does not show any significant difference (p=0.9).

It must be noted that of the 9 patients who ultimately had deficient secondary stability, 5 patients (i.e. 56%) had diaphyseal primary stability with a stem L >250 mm, versus 30% of the patients with very good/good secondary stability. However, this difference is not significant (p=0.2).

In Summary

Regarding bone stock

If the initial bone stock is deficient, some regeneration can be expected, however, it will never be very spectacular, and it is essentially possible in the absence of osteoporosis.

Moreover, in the case of deficient initial bone stock, it is often difficult to avoid a diaphyseal primary stability, which we know is less advantageous for bone regeneration.

Regarding secondary stability

An deficient initial bone stock has a rather unfavorable but not decisive impact on the secondary bone stock. A deficient initial bone stock, associated with osteoporosis, does not increase, or only by little, the risk of a deficient secondary stability, except in the case of diaphyseal primary fixation with a stem of L >250 mm.

To improve the scores of secondary bone stock and secondary stability, a surgeon can act: (1) at the time of choosing the concept and the corresponding implant (2) at the moment of choosing the strategic option and when performing the surgical procedure itself. The margin of progression of bone stock is more important, and to improve it, the regeneration of the initial bone stock should be stimulated if it is altered, or its degradation should be avoided altogether, if it is intact in the beginning.

19.1 Parameters to Choose the Right Implant

- When the press-fit concept is chosen, a stem with a *straight and tapered* configuration represents a good compromise. A *straight* shape is the best design to ensure a good surface contact and a *tapered* form has the advantage of generating a stabilizing horizontal force and a more harmonious load distribution along the contact surface bone/implant and a re-wedging is possible. These objectives are more difficult to achieve with a cylindrically-shaped stem that can create peak stresses and be the source of femoral pain.
- It must be noted that uncemented implants for revision surgery are often invasive and excessively long as it is indeed vital to ensure their primary stability! The primary drawback of these implants is a stiffening of the femur which means that the cortices are not any more submitted to constraints in traction and compression which can impede bone regeneration and entail a sharp decrease of the bone density, especially in the presence of osteoporosis. The objective is thus to select an implant that avoids such inconveniences (see Chap. 4).

19.2 Preserve or Promote the Regeneration of Bone Stock

- First, we must remember that, independent of the chosen concept, the regeneration or preservation of the bone stock is only possible if the vascularization of the cortex is assured. In this regard, one should be aware that changing the strategy during surgery, especially when preparing the anchorage zone, is always detrimental to the vascularization of the cortex. Furthermore, a surgical technique that, at first glance, can appear aggressive, is eventually often less traumatizing for the vascular environment and the bone stock. Thus, in revision, making a trochantero-diaphyscal flap to approach the femur can make it possible to overcome a number of obstacles that, in many cases, can entail a worsening of the bone stock, especially during cement removal. Moreover, if care was taken to make a pediculated flap with the vastus lateralis, this technique also has the power to stimulate bone regeneration, as already pointed out by Wagner [2] or Vives and Picault [13].
- Second, an analysis of the different factors that can have a real impact on the final result has taught us the importance of the zone of primary stability and the length of the implant, as well as taking into account the stage of osteoporosis and the extent of bone lesions that can result from a loose implant.

19.2.1 With Regard to the Femoral Approach and the Zone of Primary Stability

- If the femur is straight in the a/p plane and only slightly curved in the sagittal plane and if the bone stock is

P. Le Béguec et al., *Uncemented Femoral Stems for Revision Surgery*,
DOI 10.1007/978-3-319-03614-4_19, © Springer International Publishing Switzerland 2015

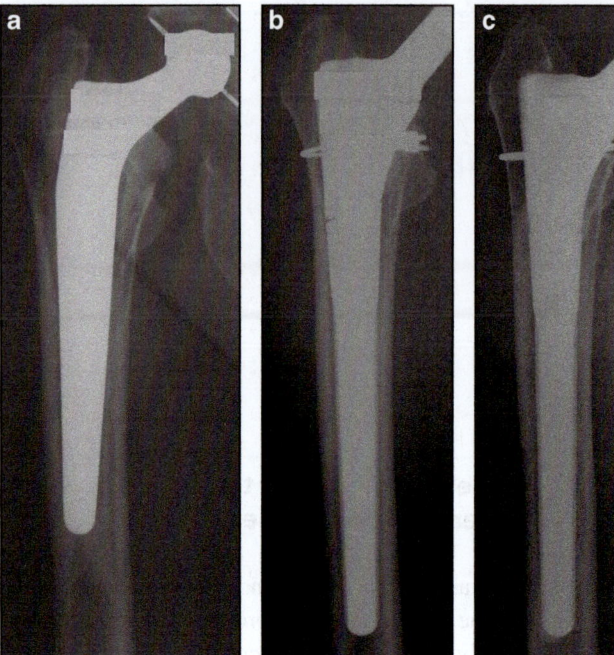

Fig. 19.1 A 65-year-old female patient, beginning osteoporosis with an average CI of 0.38 (**a**). Revision be means of an endofemoral approach with a short stem and primary fixation exclusively in the proximal region (**b**). At the 6-year follow-up, the secondary bone stock is rated as very good, 18/20 (decrease of the density in zone 1), very good osseointegration 20/20 (**c**). Global Radiographic Score: very good 20/20

preserved, proximal fixation of the implant by means of an endofemoral approach or a trochanterotomy has to be sought on principle, and, in this case, implantation of a short stem is the rule. We have noted that this is a good way to preserve the bone stock and to ensure perfect secondary stability.

- If the femur is curved, or the bone stock severely deficient, the femoral approach has to be chosen making possible a contact bone-implant in the form of a surface and, at the same time, avoid the risk of aggravating the bone stock. A pediculated trochantero-diaphyseal flap makes it possible to achieve these objectives; it also facilitates implantation of a short stem in the diaphyseal region, which is always better than selecting a long stem.

If the bone stock is severely damaged, it is also recommended to insert bone grafts or other substitutes to compensate for the loss of bone substance and to stimulate bone regeneration.

19.2.2 In the Presence of Osteoporosis

In this situation, the primary objective is to avoid overall stiffening of the femur. Thus, seeking primary stability in the proximal region of the femur must be a priority in case of osteoporosis stage 4, or even stage 3 if one wants to avoid secondary degradation of the bone stock (Fig. 19.1). Preference should be given to this option whenever possible, knowing that additional bone grafting can only be beneficial and that, under certain conditions, a trochanterotomy can make proximal fixation easier. In this situation, it is necessary to have an implant whose design makes proximal stabilization possible while avoiding fixation in the diaphyseal zone. Finally, when diaphyseal fixation is inevitable, and when implantation of a long stem with a large diameter is the only possible alternative, the choice of an uncemented concept (press-fit or fill and fit) should be thoroughly pondered and it might even be contraindicated.

Let us also recall that a confirmed osteoporosis is a surgical risk factor, especially when removing a thick cement layer that strongly adheres to weakened cortices. This is often an critical moment during surgery, and a degradation of the bone stock (via falsa, fracture) is to be feared at this stage of the intervention.

In preoperative classification, the assessment of the degree of osteoporosis is never addressed. In view of the consequences, which can sometimes be serious for the bone stock, this omission is certainly a mistake. When establishing a surgical strategy, the presence of osteoporosis must always be taken into account.

19.2.3 Promoting Osseointegration and Secondary Stability

A well osseointegrated implant will have a better chance of survival in the long term. Even if the room to maneuver is small in this area, every effort must be made to stimulate not only osseointegration and, thus, reduce the risk of loosening, but also to improve the quality of the secondary stability and, particularly, avoid an exclusively distal secondary stability.

- Even if a beneficial role can be attributed to preserving a bone stock that was rated as very good or good in the beginning, it must be noted that an improvement of the secondary bone stock is not always accompanied by an improved secondary stability, and, conversely, a deterioration of the bone stock does not mean a degradation of the secondary stability.

  The deciding factor for osseointegration and the quality of secondary stability seems to be the surgical strategy and the technique adopted by the surgeon. The beneficial role of proximal or global fixation of the implant must be remembered. And, if a flap has been made, preference must be given to a short stem and putting the cortices into contact with the implant to favor proximal osseointegration what, at the same time, reduces the risk of secondary stability solely in the distal zone of the implant. To achieve this goal, remodel the endomedullary aspect of the flap and, in a lot of cases, perform an osteotomy of the medial cortex. This surgical step, which can sometimes be laborious, requires a real effort from the surgeon... especially since this happens at the end of the surgery!

- Contrary to what has been said about bone stock, osteoporosis does not have a key role with regard to osseointegration and secondary stability. We do, however, need to question the necessity of additional bone grafting or of inserting a bone substitute, which can only be beneficial and improve secondary stability, especially if the initial bone stock is deficient (iterative loosening) and associated with an osteoporosis rated stage 3.

  An osteoinductive or osteoconductive surface treatment can facilitate secondary osseointegration, however, one needs to bear in mind that such a manufacturing characteristic does not constitute a concept that ensures the primary stability of an uncemented implant.

19.3 Complications *n = 150*

- **Secondary loosening**
  - Femoral stem: loosening in 2 cases (2%); to this number, an irreducible dislocation due to rotation of the revision stem must be added; revision with the same type of stem, but longer. In addition to these three cases, three changes of the proximal component must furthermore be added: an iterative dislocation, secondary subsidence and a fracture of the material at the site of the assembly (see below: contra-indications for a modular implant).
  - Acetabular cup: 15 cases of loosening (10%), of which 13 were revised, and 1 revision after recurrent dislocation. These acetabular failures are often the result of an inappropriate surgical technique in cases of important bone loss. It is known that in such risky situations, it is often necessary to insert extensive bone grafts and to protect these grafts with an acetabular roof ring.

- **Luxations**: 13 cases (9%)

  They were two times iterative and 1 time irreducible. In four cases, re-intervention was necessary.

  In revision surgery, dislocation remains a frequent complication, and if it is recurrent, its treatment is often delicate because there is rarely a sole cause, which is thus difficult to identify. Furthermore, based on our own results, we conclude that modularity does not seem to be efficient in the prevention of dislocation. On the other hand, a more frequent use of a double mobility cup in revision should help to reduce this high dislocation rate.

- **Bone complications**: 6 intra-operative fractures of the femur made the insertion of a longer stem necessary than originally planned, 2 cortical lyses of the flap (non-pediculated flap) and 5 secondary necroses of the greater trochanter.

  With regard to the femoral fractures, a hierarchization is necessary to differentiate between fractures that represent true complications and require additional osteosynthesis or a change of strategy, and the fractures that can be treated as simple incidents.

  No implant (straight or curved stem) can protect the surgeon from such incidents and their treatment is mainly preventive: detect and take into account a femoral curvature, even if it is not very pronounced; choose a femoral approach that enables simple and comprehensive cement removal without the risk of a fracture or a via falsa; avoid an aggressive use of the rasps or reamers, which means working within proximity of the anchorage zone; avoid long implants to reduce the risk of a fracture at the tip of the stem.

- **Infections**: 3 cases of secondary sepsis which required revision surgery for cleaning purposes, but no change of the implant. These three patients were considered as healed from their infection at the last follow-up exam.
- **Neurological complications**: a paralysis of the crural and sciatic nerve (SPE); in both cases, partial recovery. We report no vascular lesion.

19.4 Contra-indications for This Method

19.4.1 Destroyed Femoral Isthmus

These cases can occur within the framework of an iterative loosening with implantation of a long stem and extensive osteolytic lesions or within the framework of a fracture of the femur on stem. In this situation, the isthmic zone of the femur may be seriously altered, making it difficult to apply a press-fit. In such a situation, we recommend to opt for another concept: a self-locking stem finds its elective indication here, especially if the cortices are of satisfactory quality.

Reminder! A press-fit effect is not possible in the distal third of the femur.

19.4.2 Osteoporosis Stage 4

We have already pointed out the risks of severe stress shielding due to excessive stiffening of the femoral bone following the implantation of a long stem with large diameter in a severely osteoporotic femur with thinned cortices and a wide cylinder-shaped medullary canal. We believe that caution should be exercised in such conditions. If proximal fixation of the implant cannot be assured, these cases constitute a contra-indication for the press-fit concept.

In this situation, there is no doubt that extensive bone grafting is indispensible, as well as a technique type Exeter or as proposed by Kerboull [14] seem to us to be the only alternatives.

19.4.3 Risks Associated with the Assembly System of a Modular Stem

The assembly system of a modular stem is always a zone of increased fragility, and no modular implant is immune to material "failure" in this zone. In the case of the Revitan®, the rate is estimated to be 0.1%, which is an acceptable figure.

One needs to stay vigilant, however, and know the situations of risk, especially when bone destruction in the proximal femur is significant. In such a case, deficient proximal secondary osseointegration is to be feared; and in the case of an active and overweight patient, the assembly system of a modular stem is exposed to high stresses that can cause material failure. For such patients, it is often preferable to choose a monobloc implant.

The objectives of the comparative analysis of the results presented in this chapter are the following:

1. Verify whether the numerical translation of the results obtained in a qualitative assessment confirm the role previously attributed to the three so-called "impacting" factors with regard to preservation of bone stock and secondary stability.
2. Report the lessons learned by a comparative analysis of the results.

> **Warning!**
>
> Regardless of the implant or method chosen by the surgeon, it is important that every surgeon evaluates and compares his own results. Sharing experience and comparing results with those of other colleagues is enriching for all parties and an excellent means to improve performance.
>
> **By no means should such an exercise be considered an evaluation of the skills of any particular surgeon.**

20.1 Materials and Method

20.1.1 Materials

The reference group. The results of 76 consecutive revisions of total hip prostheses carried out between January 2001 and June 2004 by the same surgeon, called "Op. 1" are reported. Four patients (5%) had died from causes unrelated to the revision and were thus excluded from the study, and seven patients (9%) were lost to follow-up. Five patients (7%) were only interviewed by telephone, three of those described themselves as disabled. Ultimately, 60 hips (79%), or 58 patients, respectively (2 bilateral revisions), were included in this comparative study. There were 31 women and 27 men (27 left hips and 33 right hips). Median age was 72 years (range 49–96) and median follow-up 4.5 years (range 2–11).

The radiographic analyses and the comparative study of the results were done by the same assessor.

The results of the first 60 patients ($n = 1$–60) of the group of 150 patients served as the reference to conduct the different analyses of this work in order to constitute a homogenous group in comparison to the one whose results were evaluated (Table 20.1).

Table 20.1 Materials: general characteristics

Parameters	Reference _n 1–60_	Op. 1 _n 60_
Mean follow-up	6 Y	4.5 Y
Number (% examined)	**60** (84%)	**60** (79%)
Mean age	71 Y	72 Y
M/W (1)	23 M/35 W	27 M/31 W
Overweight (in %)	55%	60%
Revision stem	1	2
Revision cup	5	5
Femoral morphotype		
Straight	33 (55%)	27 (45%)
Curved	27 (45%)	33 (55%)
Devane classification	(_n 60_)	(_n 60_)
Manual worker, sporty	2 (3%)	1 (2%)
Light activity	0 (0%)	4 (7%)
Occasional activity	32 (53%)	22 (37%)
Semi-sedentary	25 (41%)	31 (51%)
Sedentary	2 (3%)	2 (3%)
Osteoporosis stage	(_n 60_)	(_n 60_)
St. 1 – CI: =/>0.55	6 (10%)	11 (18%)
St. 2 – CI: 0.45–0.54	23 (38%)	26 (44%)
St. 3 – CI: 0.35–0.44	21 (35%)	14 (23%)
St. 4 – CI: =/<0.34	10 (17%)	9 (15%)
Loosening stage (2)	(_n 59_)	(_n 55_)
Stage 1	14 (24%)	20 (36%)
Stage 2	16 (27%)	11 (20%)
Stage 3 A	17 (29%)	14 (25%)
Stage 3 B	11 (18%)	6 (11%)
Stage 4	1 (2%)	4 (7%)
(_1_) _Bilateral revisions_	_n 2_	_n 2_
(_2_) _Stem fracture_	_n 1_	_n 5_

P. Le Béguec et al., _Uncemented Femoral Stems for Revision Surgery_,
DOI 10.1007/978-3-319-03614-4_20, © Springer International Publishing Switzerland 2015

The comparative study of the two patient populations shows few significant differences:

1. The number of patients classified as osteoporosis stage 1 and 2 is, however, somewhat higher in the Op. 1 group than that in the reference group (62% vs 48%).
2. Stage of loosening, according to the classification of Paprosky: 58% of the patients of the reference group were classified as stage 1 and 2 in comparison to the percentage of 51% for Op. 1.

20.1.2 Method

For these two groups of patients, two evaluations, as described in the first part, were done: (1) Evaluation of the secondary bone stock (2) Evaluation of the secondary stability (weighted score).

The results are indicated as a numerical mean for each "impacting" factor (osteoporosis, initial bone stock, type of primary stability (Table 20.2). When the number of patients was smaller than 10, a grouping was made combining the cases rated as very good-good and the cases rated as average-poor. Only the differences =/> +1 point or =/< −1 point between the reference and "Op. 1" were taken into account.

An analysis of the causes that could have explained the significant difference was done.

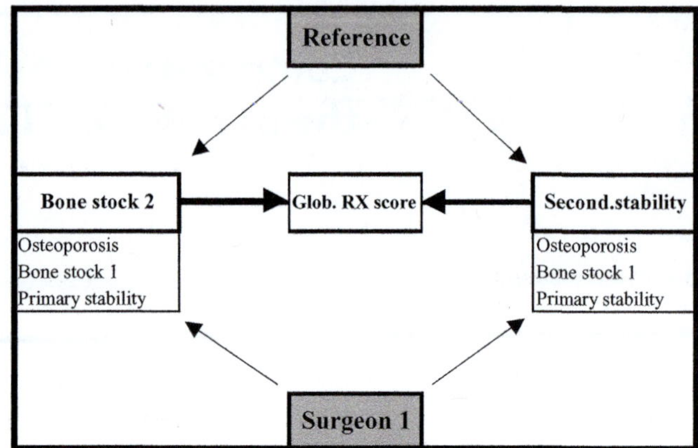

Table 20.2 Table of the method

20.2   Results

- ***Secondary bone stock*** (Table 20.3). The mean score of the reference group ($n=1$–60) and of the Op. 1 ($n=60$) is identical (13.3 points). For the reference group, there is a non-significant regression of −0.9 points of the value of the initial bone stock (13.3 vs 14.2) (p=0.6) and of −0.2 points (13.5 vs 13.3) for the Op. 1 (p=0.4). The evolution between initial and secondary bone stock is not statistically different from one surgeon to another (p=0.3).
- ***Secondary stability*** (weighted score) (Table 20.4). The mean score of the reference group ($n=1$–60) and of the Op. 1 ($n=60$) shows a difference of **−1.6 points** to the disadvantage of the Op. 1 (15.9 vs 14.3) (non-significant limit, p=0.07).

Table 20.3 Results secondary bone stock

Second. bone stock	Ref. (*n* 1–60)		Op.1 (*n* 60)		Difference	
Mean score	**13.3**		**13.3**		**0**	
Osteoporosis						
St.1: Very good	*n 6* **19.0**	*n 29 16*	*n 11* **16.3**	*n 37 15*	**−2.7**	*−1*
St.2: Good	*n 23* **15.2**		*n 26* **14.5**		**−0.7**	
St.3: Average	*n 21* **12.5**	*n 31 10.7*	*n 14* **11.8**	*n 23 10.4*	**−0.7**	*−0.3*
St.4: Poor	*n 10* **7.0**		*n 9* **8.2**		**+1.2**	
Bone stock 1	**14.2**		**13.5**			
Very good	*n 18* **16.2**	*n 39 15*	*n 8* **16.2**	*n 35 14.4*	**0**	*−0.6*
Good	*n 21* **14.0**		*n 27* **13.9**		**−0.1**	
Average	*n 15* **11.2**	*n 21 10*	*n 20* **12.5**	*n 25 11.7*	**+1.3**	*+1.7*
Poor	*n 6* **7.0**		*n 5* **8.4**		**+1.4**	
Primary stability						
Proximal	*n 10* **15.6**	/	/	/	/	/
Global	*n 10* **13.6**		/		/	
Diaphyseal	*n 26* **11.2**	/	*n 42* **13.7**	/	**+2.5**	/
3-point	*n 14* **15.3**		*n 18* **12.3**		**−3**	

Table 20.4 Results secondary stability

Secondary stability	Ref. (*n* 1–60)		Op.1 (*n* 60)		Difference	
Mean score	**15.9**		**14.3**		**–1.6**	
Osteoporosis						
St.1: Very good	*n 6* **16.3**	*n 29* **16.6**	*n 11* **14.8**	*n 37* **14.1**	**–15**	**–2.5**
St.2: Good	*n 23* **16.7**		*n 26* **13.8**		**–2.9**	
St.3: Average	*n 21* **14.8**	*n 31* **15.1**	*n 14* **15.1**	*n 23* **14.6**	**+0.3**	**–0.5**
St.4: Poor	*n 10* **15.8**		*n 9* **14.0**		**–1.8**	
Bone stock 1						
Very good	*n 18* **18.4**	*n 39* **17**	*n 8* **14.7**	*n 35* **13.6**	**3.7**	**–3.4**
Good	*n 21* **15.7**		*n 27* **13.3**		**–2.4**	
Average	*n 15* **13.8**	*n 21* **13.8**	*n 20* **15.3**	*n 25* **15.3**	**+ 1.5**	**+1.5**
Poor	*n 6* **14.0**		*n 5* **15.2**		**+ 1.2**	
Primary stability						
Proximal	*n 10* **18.1**	/	/	/	/	/
Global	*n 10* **17.4**		/		/	
Diaphyseal	*n 26* **14.4**	/	*n 42* **14.5**	/	**+0.1**	/
3-point	*n 14* **15.9**		*n 18* **14.0**		**–1.9**	

20.2.1 Differences Depending on the Stage of Osteoporosis

The reported discrepancies pertain to bone stock and secondary stability, and only osteoporosis stages **1 and 2** are implicated.

20.2.1.1 Secondary Bone Stock: Difference of –1 Point to the Disadvantage Op. 1
(Tables 20.3 and 20.5)

- This difference, to the disadvantage of Op. 1, yet not significant (p=0.3), cannot be explained by a more frequent impairment of the initial bone stock in the group of Op. 1 (32% vs 17%) because we have observed that, in the absence of osteoporosis (which is the case here), an improvement of a deficient initial bone stock is often possible.
- The reason for this discrepancy is more likely to be attributed to the type of diaphyseal primary stability, which is, overall, less favorable for the secondary bone stock.

  In the group Op. 1, 28 of the 37 cases (i.e. 76%) had this type of primary stability, versus 9 cases of the 29 cases (i.e. 31%) in the reference group, which is significant (p<0.0001).

Table 20.5 Osteoporosis St. 1 and 2. Impact of initial bone stock and type primary stability on secondary bone stock and secondary stability

Bone stock 1	VG	G	Av	P
Ref. *n=29*	11	13	4	1
Op. 1 *n=37*	7	18	11	1
Stability 1	**Prox.**	**Glob.**	**Diaph.**	**3-point**
Ref. *n=29*	6	7	9	7
Op.1 *n=37*	/	/	28	9

20.2.1.2 Secondary Stability: Difference –2.5 Points to the Disadvantage of Op. 1 (Tables 20.4 and 20.5)

- This discrepancy, which is significant and to the disadvantage of Op. 1, finds its first explanation in the frequent, however not significant, impairment of the initial bone stock in the group of Op. 1 (p=0.2). We have observed that an initial bone stock, evaluated as average-poor is less favorable for secondary stability.
- Another explanation lies in the proximal stabilization of the implant, whose beneficial role for secondary stability has been discussed: none patient of the Op.1 benefited of a primary proximal or global fixation.

20.2.2 Differences Depending on the Value of the Initial Bone Stock

This concerns the four stages of the value of the initial bone stock.

20.2.2.1 Initial Bone Stock Very Good-Good

The difference only applies to secondary stability: 3.4 points to the disadvantage of Op. 1 (Tables 20.4 and 20.6)

- This difference, significantly to the disadvantage (p=0.002) of Op. 1, does not find its explanation in the degree of osteoporosis, estimated VG-G in 62% of the cases in the reference group and in 71% of the cases in the series of Op. 1 (non-significant p=0.4) and which, does not have a decisive impact on secondary stability.
- The cause of this deficit is to be found in the type primary stability which is of type diaphyseal for 77% of the

Table 20.6 Initial bone stock VG-G. Impact of osteoporosis and type primary stability on secondary stability

Osteoporosis	St.1: VG	St.2: G	St.3: Av	St.4: P
Ref. *n=39*	6	18	10	5
Op.1 *n=35*	7	18	6	4
Stability 1	Prox.	Glob.	Diaph.	3-point
Ref. *n=39*	9	9	13	8
Op.1 *n=35*	/	/	27	8

cases in the Op. 1 versus 33% in the reference group (significant difference p<0.0001) and this type of primary stability is known to be less favorable for secondary stability.

On the contrary, primary stability of type proximal and global which are known to be favorable to osseointegration and secondary stability were achieved in 46% of the cases in the reference series and in none of the cases in the Op. 1 group (p=0.002).

20.2.2.2 Initial Bone Stock Average-Poor

The differences concern both, secondary bone stock and secondary stability.

1. Secondary bone stock: difference +1.7 points to the advantage of Op. 1 (Tables 20.3 and 20.7)
- This difference, to the advantage of Op. 1, which is, however, not significant (p=0.3), was helped by the increased presence of an osteoporosis assessed as average-poor in the reference group: 76% of the cases versus 52% of the cases in the series of Op. 1 (non-significant trend p=0.09). We have seen that the presence of osteoporosis is not favorable to bone regeneration.

Table 20.7 Initial bone stock Av-P. Impact of osteoporosis and type primary stability on secondary bone stock and secondary stability

Osteoporosis	St.1:VG	St.2: G	St.3: Av	St.4: P
Ref. *n=21*	/	5	11	5
Op.1 *n=25*	4	8	8	5
Stability 1	Prox.	Glob.	Diaph.	3-point
Ref. *n=21*	1	1	13	6
Op. 1 *n=25*	/	/	15	10

- Also the rather negative impact on secondary bone stock of a stem length >200 mm with diaphyseal fixation must be noted. This situation was encountered in 92% of the cases in the reference series and in 33% in the Op. 1 series, which constitutes a significant difference p=0.001.

2. Secondary stability: difference +1.5 points to the advantage Op. 1 (Tables 20.4 and 20.7)
- This difference, not significantly to the advantage of Op. 1 (p=0.3), can only be partially explained by the higher incidence of osteoporosis rated as average-poor in the reference series (76% vs 52% for Op. 1). We have observed that the association of osteoporosis and a deficient initial bone stock (which is the case here) does not have a particularly unfavorable impact on secondary stability.
- A more certain explanation can be found in the length of the implant in the case of diaphyseal primary stability. In the reference series, 10 of the 13 cases (i.e. 77%) had a so-called long diaphyseal primary stability with a stem length of >250 mm; on the other hand, in the 15 patients of Op. 1 which are in the same situation, no implant exceeds 250 mm and in all cases, the stability was diaphyseal and can be described as short. We have noted that a so-called long diaphyseal primary stability is the least favorable for secondary stability.

20.2.3 Differences Depending on the Type of Primary Stability

20.2.3.1 Diaphyseal Primary Stability

The difference only applies to secondary bone stock: +2.5 points to the advantage of Op. 1 (Tables 20.3 and 20.8)
- This difference, to the advantage of Op. 1, yet not significant (p=0.1), can be attributed to the significantly higher number of cases of osteoporosis rated as very good/good in the series of Op. 1, which is favorable for secondary bone stock: 67% in the series of Op. 1 versus 35% for the reference group (p=0.009).

Table 20.8 Diaphyseal primary stability. Impact of osteoporosis and initial bone stock on secondary bone stock

Osteoporosis	St.1: VG	St.2: G	St.3: Av	St.4: P
Ref. *n=26*	1	8	10	7
Op.1 *n=42*	7	21	10	4
Bone stock 1	VG	G	Av	P
Ref. *n=26*	3	10	8	5
Op. 1 *n=42*	7	20	13	2

- Also to be noted in the series of Op. 1 is a smaller and non-significant incidence (p=0.2) of deficient initial bone stock (36% versus 50% for the reference series) and the more frequent use of a short stem, which is known to be less unfavorable for the bone stock (significant p<0.0001).

20.2.3.2 3-Point Primary Stability

The differences apply to both, secondary bone stock as well as secondary stability.

1. Secondary Bone Stock: Difference −3 Points to the Disadvantage of Op. 1 (Table 20.3 and 20.9)

- This difference, which is borderline significant (p=0.06), can be explained by the presence in the series of Op. 1 of osteoporosis stage 4 in 5 cases (i.e. 28%) , while there is none in the reference group (p=0.05) (qualitative test poor versus very good-good versus average). It is known that osteoporosis stage 4 is very unfavorable for the bone stock.

Table 20.9 3-point stability. Impact of osteoporosis and initial bone stock on secondary bone stock and secondary stability

Osteoporosis	St.1:VG	St.2: G	St.3: Av	St.4: P
Ref. $n=14$	2	5	7	0
Op.1 $n=18$	4	5	4	5
Bone stock 1	VG	G	Av	P
Ref. $n=14$	3	5	5	1
Op.1 $n=18$	1	7	7	3

2. Secondary Stability: Difference −1.9 Points to the Disadvantage of Op. 1 (Table 20.4 and 20.9)

To explain this discrepancy, which is not significant (p=0.2) but to the disadvantage of Op. 1, we can incriminate a more frequent deficiency of the initial bone stock, 56% in the Op. 1 group versus 43% in the reference group (not significant p=0.5). It is probably also necessary to evoke the femoral approach knowing that, within the framework of a 3 points support, a endofemoral approach (performed in 76% of the cases to the reference) is more favorable for the secondary stability than a femoral flap performed in 89% of the cases to Op. 1 (16.2 vs 14 points in numerical value).

20.3 Discussion-Conclusions

20.3.1 The Global Score

The discrepancy of **−0.9 points**, to the disadvantage of Op. 1 (14.7 versus 13.8), yet not significant (p=0.3), is the result, in a qualitative assessment, of a decrease of the cases rated as very good and in an increase of the cases rated as average in the Op. 1 group (Table 20.10).

This discrepancy is only due to less good results of the secondary stability in the Op. 1 group (difference of −1.6 points) (p=0.07 borderline significant), and, ultimately, it seems logical when considering that secondary stability only counts for half in the final global result.

Table 20.10 Comparison of global scores

Global score		Very good	Good	Average	Poor
Reference	Number %	12 (20%)	23 (38%)	12 (20%)	13 (22%)
$n=60$	Num. value	20	16.8	12.4	8.3
Op. 1	Number %	6 (10%)	23 (38%)	17 (29%)	14 (23%)
$n=60$	Num. value	20	16.7	12.6	7.8

20.3.2 Numerical Translation of the Results

- The numerical translation of a result given in qualitative version allows quantification of a difference and serves primarily to identify the factors that can have a real influence – positive or negative – on the final result.
- The progressive decrease of the numerical values gathered from the analysis of the results of the degree of osteoporosis and the value of the initial bone stock, especially in the reference group, tends to validate the hierarchization of the criteria defined to qualify the different stages of these two factors.
- The numerical translation of the global score is logical and shows a significant difference between the different qualitative stages, which was the desired objective (Table 20.10).
- With regard to the impacting factors, the comparison of the results of the two groups of patients, especially the numerical results, confirms the role of osteoporosis, deficient initial bone stock and the type of primary stability (length of the implant and proximal stabilization) in the preservation or regeneration of secondary bone stock and secondary stability.

20.3.3 Comparative Analysis of the Results

20.3.3.1 Secondary Bone Stock

The fact that there is no difference between the two groups that were studied reminds us that: (1) a lack of experience in the beginning of the learning curve is not favorable for secondary bone stock (2) this is the main parameter where it pays to be vigilant if one wants to improve the overall result (bone stock and secondary stability).

To explain the regression of −0.9 points of the value of the initial bone stock for the reference group and of −0.2 points for the Op. 1, the negative impact of a surgery, which was probably somewhat more aggressive in the beginning of the learning curve, on the bone vascularization cannot be excluded and also making a non-pediculated flap, which was the case in 35% (21 patients) of the cases in the reference series.

20.3.3.2 Secondary Stability (Weighted Score)

To explain the deficient situations in the Op. 1 group in comparison to the reference group, only the strategic choice and the surgical procedure itself can be blamed.

- Firstly, with regard to the strategic choice, the absence of primary global or proximal stability must be pointed out. It is known that these fixation methods are favorable for osseointegration and that a proximal primary stability makes it possible to prevent severe degradation of the bone stock in osteoporotic conditions. It is probable that these types of primary fixation could (or should) have been indicated in some of the 27 patients that had a straight femoral morphotype in the beginning!

- Secondly, a unambiguous strategic choice to the Op. 1, i.e. making a femoral approach by means of a trochantero-diaphyseal flap, automatically implies a primary stability in the diaphyseal region, which is, overall, less favorable for secondary stability, especially if, after making a flap, proximal stabilization is not achieved whenever possible. We have observed that this was more often the case in the group of the Op. 1.

Furthermore, we cannot exclude that a femoral flap can have, in itself, a role rather negative for the osseointegration and the secondary stability.

Finally, this comparative analysis clearly confirms the importance of the choice of the surgical strategy (femoral approach and zone of primary stability) and the surgical technique, especially in revision surgery.

1. Overview table of the "impacting" factors

	Secondary bone stock			Secondary stability		
Osteoporosis	+	+/-	-	+	+/-	-
Very good	■				■	
Good	■				■	
Average		■			■	
Poor (1)			■	■		
Bone stock 1	+	+/-	-	+	+/-	-
Very good	■				■	
Good	■				■	
Average		■			■	
Poor			■		■	
Primary stab.	+	+/-	-	+	+/-	-
Proximal (2)	■			■		
Global (3)		■		■		
Dia. Short (4)		■			■	
Dia. long			■			■
3-points		■			■	

● Positive impact ● Variable impact ● Negative impact

1. Impact – or bone stock and + for secondary stability by means of a stress shielding
2. Proximal primary stability helps to avoid significant degradation, particularly when the initial bone stock is good or very good or in cases fo osteoporosis.
3. Global primary stability can promote stress shielding +/ in certain situations.
4. Negative impact on bone stock, especially in case of osteoporosis, and on secondary bone stock if no proximal stabilization of the implant

2. Value secondary bone stock

According to type of primary stability, value of initial bone stock and degree of osteoporosis

Type of primary stability		Prox.	Global	Dia. short	Dia. long	3-point
Initial hone stock; VG/G **CI: VG/G (no osteoporosis)** *n=63*		*n=6*	*n=11*	*n=22*	*n=9*	*n=15*
n=8 (13 %)	**VG** *n=41*	2	5	15	6	13
	G *n=14*	3	5	4	1	1
	Av *n=8*	1	1	3	2	1
	P *n=0*	/	/	/	/	/
Initial bone stock: Av/P **CI: VG/G (no osteoporosis)** *n=13*		*n=1*	*n=0*	*n=6*	*n=2*	*n=4*
n=2 (15 %)	**VG** *n=4*	/	/	2	1	1
	G *n=7*	1	/	2	1	3
	Av *n=1*	/	/	1	/	/
	P *n=1*	/	/	1	/	/
Initial bone stock: VG/G **C1: Av/P (osteoporosis)** *n=42*		*n=6*	*n=5*	*n=13*	*n=10*	*n=8*
n=21 (50 %)	**TB** *n=15*	4	1	2	4	4
	B *n=6*	/	1	3	1	1
	My *n=11*	1	2	4	2	2
	Mv *n=10*	1	1	4	3	1
Initial hone stock: Av/P **CI: Av/P (osteoporosis)** *n=32*		*n=0*	*n=1*	*n=8*	*n=12*	*n=11*
n=19 (59 %)	**VG** *n=6*	/	/	2	3	1
	G *n=7*	/	/	1	2	4
	Av *n=7*	/	/	2	1	4
	P *n=12*	/	1	3	6	2

CI cortical index

1. The presence of osteoporosis is the factor with the highest negative impact on the regeneration of bone stock.
2. A deficient initial bone stock does not have a particularly negative effect on bone regeneration in the absence of osteoporosis.
3. Diaphyseal primary stability if the least favorable for bone regeneration, especially in the presence of osteoporosis.
4. The association of the presence of osteoporosis+deficient initial bone stock and diaphyseal primary stability with a long stem have a particularly negative impact on the secondary bone stock.

3. Value secondary stability

According to type of primary stability, value of initial bone stock and degree of osteoporosis

Type of primary stability		Prox	Global.	Dia. short	Dia. long	3-point
Initial bone stock; VG/G **CI: VG/G (no osteoporosis)** *n=63*		*n=6*	*n=11*	*n=22*	*n=9*	*n=15*
n=7 (11 %)	**VG** *n=39*	5	7	11	6	10
	G *n=17*	1	4	6	2	4
	Av *n=5*	/	/	4	1	/
	P *n=2*	/	/	1	1	1
Initial bone stock: Av/P **CI: VG/G (no osteoporosis)** *n=13*		*n=1*	*n=0*	*n=6*	*n=2*	*n=4*
n=4 (31 %)	**VG** *n=5*	/	/	3	I	2
	G *n=4*	1	1	1	1	2
	Av *n=4*	1	/	2	1	/
	P *n=0*	/	/	/	/	/
Initial bone stock: VG/G **CI: Av/P (osteoporosis)** *n=42*		*n=6*	*n=5*	*n=13*	*n=10*	*n=8*
n=6 (14 %)	**VG** *n=25*	6	5	8	2	4
	G *n=11*	/	/	2	6	3
	Av *n=4*	/	/	1	2	1
	P *n=2*	/	/	2	/	/
Initial bone stock: AV/P **CI: Av/P (osteoporosis)** *n=32*		*n=0*	*n=1*	*n=8*	*n=12*	*n=11*
n=9 (28 %)	**VG** *n=14*	/	/	6	4	4
	G *n=9*	/	1	1	3	4
	Av *n=6*	/	/	1	3	2
	P *n=3*	/	/	/	2	1

CI cortical index

1. A deficient initial bone stock has a rather unfavorable impact on secondary stability.
2. Osteoporosis as such is not a particularly negative factor for secondary stability.
3. Diaphyseal primary stability is the least favorable for secondary stability.
4. The negative impact of a diaphyseal or so-called long primary stability (stem L. >250 mm), in combination with an osteoporosis and a deficient initial bone stock, must be pointed out.

Uncemented Femoral Stems for Revision Surgery

The Press-fit Concept - Planning - Surgical Technique - Evaluation

Pierre Le Béguec • François Canovas • Olivier Roche • Mathias Goldschild • Julien Batard

ISBN 978-3-319-03613-7
ISBN 978-3-319-03614-4 (eBook)
DOI 10.1007/978-3-319-03614-4

Some errors occurred in the present version of the book:

Erratum to:
Chapter 12 in: P. Le Béguec et al., Uncemented Femoral Stems for Revision Surgery,
DOI 10.1007/978-3-319-03614-4_12, © Springer International Publishing Switzerland 2015

– Tables 12.1 et 12.4: read "**3a** Diaphyseal stability" instead of "**3a** Dispheal stability"

– Captions:
  • Fig. 12.7, 12.8: read "diaphyseal" instead of "distal +"

The online version of the original book can be found at:
DOI 10.1007/978-3-319-03614-4_12
DOI 10.1007/978-3-319-03614-4_13
DOI 10.1007/978-3-319-03614-4_16
DOI 10.1007/978-3-319-03614-4_17
DOI 10.1007/978-3-319-03614-4_18

Erratum to:
Chapter 13 in: P. Le Béguec et al., Uncemented Femoral Stems for Revision Surgery,
DOI 10.1007/978-3-319-03614-4_13, © Springer International Publishing Switzerland 2015

– Captions:
  • Fig. 13.4: read "diaphyseal" instead of "distal +"

Erratum to:
Chapter 16 in: P. Le Béguec et al., Uncemented Femoral Stems for Revision Surgery,
DOI 10.1007/978-3-319-03614-4_16, © Springer International Publishing Switzerland 2015

– Captions:
  • Fig. 16.8: read "diaphyseal" instead of "distal +"

Erratum to:
Chapter 17 in: P. Le Béguec et al., Uncemented Femoral Stems for Revision Surgery,
DOI 10.1007/978-3-319-03614-4_17, © Springer International Publishing Switzerland 2015

– Page 108: Fig. 17.3 X-ray have to be replaced by Fig. 17.4 X-ray and vice versa

– Captions:
  • Fig. 17.3: read "Diaphyseal stability" instead of "Distal secondary stability+"

Erratum to:
Chapter 18 in: P. Le Béguec et al., Uncemented Femoral Stems for Revision Surgery,
DOI 10.1007/978-3-319-03614-4_18, © Springer International Publishing Switzerland 2015

– Captions:
  • Fig. 18.1: read "diaphyseal" instead of "distal +"

The following explanations are part of the Front Matter of the Part "Evaluation of Radiographic Results – How?"

To perform well, a surgeon has to select a "good" prosthesis and have access to all information that enables him to use the chosen implant well.

Yet, this is not sufficient. The surgeon must also be able to improve his own results; he can only meet this challenge if he has a reliable and rigorous radiological method of analysis to appreciate a result as a whole.

A result can be qualified as "good" only if it is rated as such from both, a clinical and radiological perspective. Current methods proposed for the clinical evaluation of hip prostheses, such as the Harris (HHS) [16] and Merle d'Aubigné-Postel (MAP) [17] scores, are admitted and used by most experts. The same is not true for the radiographic evaluation of uncemented femoral stems.

Radiographic evaluation - how?

The methods recommended by Engh and al in 1990 [18], or by Epinette and al in 1994 [19], concern uncemented femoral stems for primary surgery and are still relevant today. The only objective of these methods is an evaluation of osseointegration and secondary stability, which is insufficient, especially within the framework of a revision, where the quality of the bone stock is not taken into account. The classification for stress shielding proposed by Engh and al [20], usually used to this end, does not mitigate this lack. This method is not adapted for revisions. In particular, it does not evaluate all bone modifications that can arise in the case of an uncemented revision stem. Boisgard and al [21] have published a method which evaluates the femoral bone stock, but it does not take into account osseo-integration and/or the stability of the implant.

To our knowledge, no method of radiographic evaluation addresses the double objective which consists in evaluating at the same time the quality of the bone stock surrounding an uncemented prosthesis as well as the quality of osseointegration and secondary stability of a primary or revision stem. This is surprising considering that there is not always a narrow relation between a clinical and a radiographic result. To gain a clear idea of the value of an implant and of a surgical method, the radiographic analysis remains the only instrument that provides objective results!

Radiographic evaluation - why?

- Firstly, a rigorous radiographic evaluation yielding a comprehensive result is a good means to choose an implant in reasoned manner. While many prostheses provide good immediate results, it is not of the same in the long term. In the case of uncemented femoral prostheses, a stem which ensures large filling of the medullary cavity illustrates this well. Achieving primary stability and a pain-free hip with such implants is easy; yet, after several

years, the risk of a degradation of the bone stock around the implant is considerable and can make a new intervention risky.

Using a well designed prosthesis to ensure reliable primary stability while protecting the bone stock is today's challenge when selecting an uncemented femoral prosthesis.

- Secondly, the radiographic evaluation serves as a good means to know which directions must be followed to improve a result. When choosing an uncemented stem, it is possible to intervene in several ways : when selecting the surgical strategy and during the actual surgery; by taking into account the presence of osteoporosis as well as the extent of bone defects resulting from a loosened stem in revision surgery.

Materials

To validate the evaluation method proposed below, we refer to a retrospective study based on 183 consecutive THA revisions (175 patients) performed between April 1996 and December 2000. All patients had an implanted prosthesis at the time of revision. Ten patients (6%) who had died for reasons unrelated to revision surgery were excluded and 6 patients (3%) were lost to follow up. Seventeen patients (9%) were only interviewed by telephone. None of these patients had undergone additional surgery, and all had a satisfactory autonomy without inguinal or femoral pain.

A total of 150 hip replacements (82%), corresponding to 142 patients, were evaluated in this study (8 bilateral revisions). There were 78 women and 72 men (59 left hips and 91 right hips). Mean age was 69 years (27-89) and average follow-up was 6 years (2-15). All operations were performed by the senior surgeon (LBP), and the patients were reviewed by an independent observer (MG). The surgical approach was anterolateral in 26 cases and posterolateral in 124 cases. The femoral approach was exclusively endofemoral in 38 cases, by trochanteric osteotomy in 8 cases, and in 104 cases, an extended femoral osteotomy was performed.

The femoral prosthesis implanted was a straight uncemented stem, tapered and modular, made from a titanium alloy with a rough-blasted surface (Revitan®, Zimmer GmbH, Winterthur, Switzerland). Primary stability is obtained by press-fit over a distance of about 3 cm. No bone graft was used. During a postoperative period of 2 weeks, partial weight-bearing, using two crutches, was allowed.

The necessary radiographs

- We have voluntarily limited the number of radiographs necessary for performing the analysis proposed in this study to three a/p views: an anteroposterior (AP) X-ray of the femur taken immediately after revision surgery and two AP X-rays taken during the last follow-up visit (a minimum follow-up of two years is necessary): one classic and one negative X-ray. The radiographic reproducibility was assessed according to the criteria defined by Tannast and al [22].

- To assess bone density, we use the possibilities offered by the digitalization of radiographs which allows a comparison of the intensity of the grey levels on two successive radiographs, one being made immediately after surgery and the other at the time of the last follow-up. A decrease of the bone density is rated as "moderate" when the ratio is lower than 50 % when compared to the reference value, and "severe" when the ratio is superior to 50 % (see appendix 2).

To assess bone density, we use the possibilities offered by the digitalization of radiographs which allows a comparison of the intensity of the grey levels on two successive radiographs, one being made immediately after surgery and the other at the time of the last follow-up. A decrease of the bone density is rated as "moderate" when the ratio is lower than 50 % when compared to the reference value, and "severe" when the ratio is superior to 50 % (see appendix 2).

NB. We are fully aware that this study would be more complete with a radiographic evaluation in the sagittal plane. We estimate, however, that would not be realistic as it is difficult to obtain suitable radiographs in this plane in all cases. As for the more sophisticated examinations (scanner, studies of bone densitometry), they are usually reserved for more targeted evaluations and for short series.

IT technology

- IT is particularly useful at the time of collection of clinical and radiological data (see appendix 3). It can also useful to automatically generate the value of the Global Radiological Score (GRS) which is the synthesis of two evaluations made beforehand.
- A computing system is essential for the calculation of secondary subsidence and, especially, to measure the thickness of the cortices (cortical index : CI). This objective data can help in the assessment of the degree of preoperative osteoporosis and in the evaluation of bone remodeling around an uncemented implant. All our evaluations were performed with the EvalNet Software (LeadTools®, Lead Technologies, Inc. Charlotte, NC, USA).

NB: To evaluate bone stock, measuring the cortical thickness is questionable within the framework of a revision, except in cases of cortical atrophy with a decrease of bone density. Indeed, to obtain a meaningful value, the measures must be made based on a fixed point and/or a distance from a point of reference that remains always the same. In the case of revision, it is difficult to choose the zone of the femur which must be measured in advance. This zone can vary from one patient to another. Depending on the circumstances, this measure can be abnormally favorable or unfavorable, and not reflect the overall quality of the femoral cortices well.

Statistical analysis

The statistical analysis was done with the statistical software SAS (version 9.3; SAS Institute; Cary, NC).

The qualitative variables are expressed in actual numbers and percentages, continues variables in the form of mean values. Independence tests between two qualitative variables in non-linked series were done by means of a Chi2 test (or Fisher's exact test, if necessary).

The search for associations between initial and secondary bone stock was done with the Chi2 test by Mac Nemar.

The comparison of the quantitative variables between the different groups was done with the non-parametric Wilcoxon test because of the non-normality of the distribution of the numbers.

The inter- and intra-observer reproducibility was quantified with the help of the intra-class correlation coefficient (Fleiss type 2) with a confidence interval of 95% [23]. The agreement between the discretized results of the scores was measured by means of the Kappa coefficient with a confidence interval of 95%.

For the validity study, a correlation with the Engh score was measured with the help of Spearman's non-parametric correlation coefficient with a confidence interval of 95%.

The materiality threshold is 5% (i.e. a value of 0.05) and, unless otherwise specified in the text, the statistics based on the variables that include the modalities: Very good / Good / Average / Poor were done by systematically allocating them into the groups "Very good and good" versus "Average and poor".

General Conclusions

What You Should!

1. Prior to surgery, have at your disposal appropriate radiographs (in number and quality) to undertake a rigorous radiographic analysis and choose the right strategy taking into account the requirements imposed by the press-fit concept.
2. Take into account the presence of a femoral curvature and an osteoporosis when choosing your strategy.
3. Do not hesitate to choose a femoral approach by means of a pediculated lateral trochantero-diaphyseal flap, especially when the femur is curved – even in the absence of bone defects!
4. Remove all cement without aggravating bony lesions. This requires a perfect vision of the endomedullary space.
5. Prepare the anchorage area with rasps or reamers only when you are sure that you are working in a straight segment of the femur and after having removed all extramedullary (greater trochanter) and intra-medullary (cement) obstacles.
6. When an endofemoral approach has been chosen, make a wide opening of the greater trochanter and seek proximal fixation in the metaphyseo-diaphyseal zone. Only seek diaphyseal fixation if proximal fixation is not possible.
    - In a first step, prepare the implantation area with rasps (if a diaphyseal fixation is necessary, use the reamers).
    - Select the implant with the rasp that also serves as trial prosthesis.
    - Use the modularity of the rasp wisely during the two surgical steps (preparation and choice of implant).
    - Select the final implant after performing one or several trial reductions and retain a safety margin by making the trial reductions with a medium neck length.
    - Insert the final implant in one step after assembling the two prosthetic components outside the femur in the case of a modular implant.
7. When a trochantero-diaphyseal flap has been chosen, the fixation of the implant can only be diaphyseal. In this situation, the reamers are only used to make the medullary cavity tapered, not to select the implant, which is done with the trial prosthesis.
    - Use the tapered zone of the implant to ensure primary stability and keep a conical reserve for wedging. To do this, preference should be given to the implant diameter rather than its length, which means that often a shorter stem should be chosen.
    - Select the implant with the help of a modular trial prosthesis (for the Revitan® system: avoid choosing an extreme proximal component of a length of 95 or 105 mm) and choose a medium neck for the trial reduction to keep a margin of maneuver when inserting the final implant.
    - Insert the final implant as a monobloc component that wedges at the right level if the preparation of the anchorage zone and the selection of the implant have been done carefully (in this case, the assembly of the two prosthetic components can be done outside the femur).
    - If the final stem is modular, it is possible to perform an implantation in two steps. In this case, the assembly of the two prosthetic components can be done in situ.
8. If a femoral flap was performed, reposition it carefully, especially, if the fixation in the diaphyseal region is somewhat precarious, and apply a cerclage wire in the form a tension band if the greater trochanter is fragile.
9. With regard to the postoperative protocol, avoid giving ambiguous instructions and, if full weight-bearing is not possible or constitutes a risk, it is preferable to keep the patient under surveillance during the period of partial weight-bearing.

What You Should Not!

1. Begin surgery without having at your disposal a radiographic evaluation that makes it possible to identify the main obstacles to the implantation of a straight press-fit stem, especially the presence of a femoral curvature.

P. Le Béguec et al., *Uncemented Femoral Stems for Revision Surgery*,
DOI 10.1007/978-3-319-03614-4, © Springer International Publishing Switzerland 2015

2. Think that all the cement can be removed without difficulty and without aggravating bone lesions when the cortices are weakened (granulomas, stress shielding, osteoporosis). In such a situation, there is a risk of incomplete cement removal or a via falsa, or even of a fracture.

3. Persist in wanting to implant a straight stem in a curved femur using an endofemoral approach when a femorotomy by means of a lateral trochantero-diaphyseal flap, associated with an osteotomy of the medial cortex, is always necessary in these cases.

4. Think that a femoral curvature can be reduced with the help of a tapered reamer

5. Achieve a diaphyseal press-fit effect with a long stem by only an endofemoral approach because this means taking the risk of 3-point support and of poor wedging. It is always easier to achieve a good press-fit effect (surface contact and wedging) with a short stem, especially if we are near of the anchorage zone.

6. Choose an implant on the basis of the references indicated on the reamer because this implies that an implant longer than necessary is selected in many cases.

7. Not keeping a safety margin when choosing the neck length (or, more rarely, when selecting the length of the final proximal component in the case of a modular prosthesis) means running the risk of insufficient wedging when inserting the final stem.

8. Wanting to assemble the components in situ when an endofemoral approach was chosen.

9. Impact the trial prosthesis or the final implant with heavy hammer blows and without controlling progression or continue to impact the component deeper if its progression has come to a halt. This means running the risk of a fracture or hemming of the prosthesis.

10. Let the patient return home before weight-bearing is authorized.

Table Radiographic Score

Postoperative bone stock: 1- immediate 2- secondary

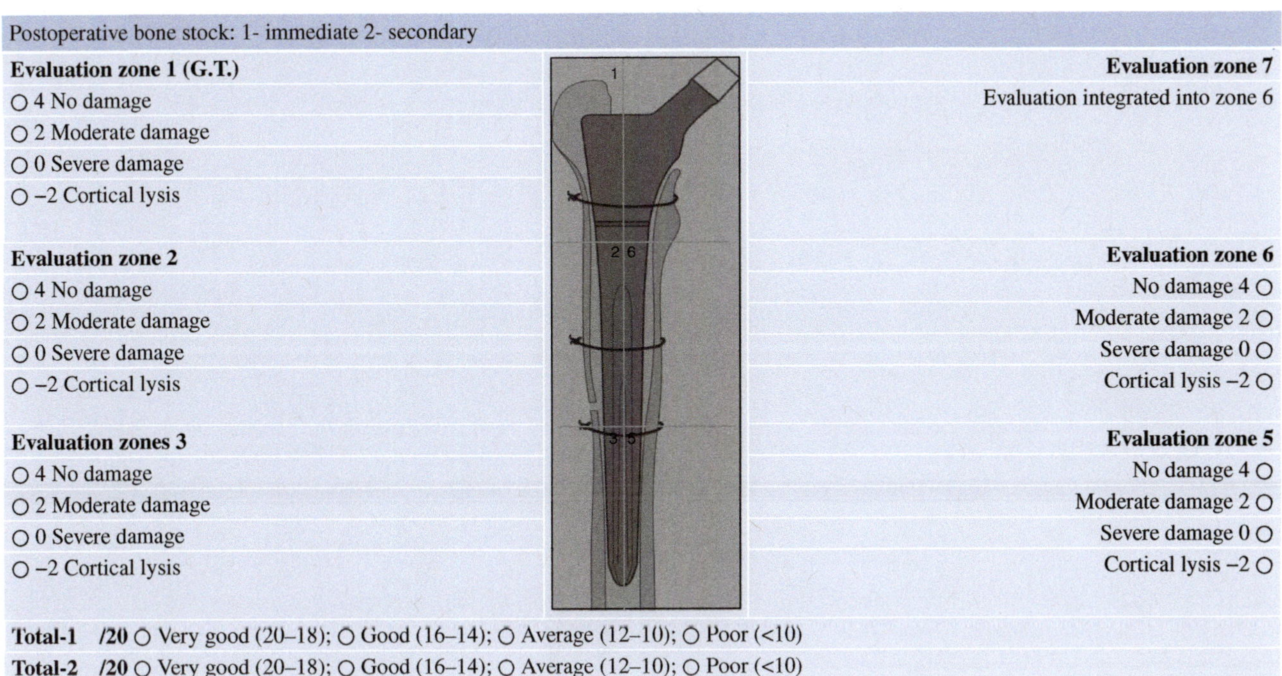

Evaluation zone 1 (G.T.)	Evaluation zone 7
○ 4 No damage	Evaluation integrated into zone 6
○ 2 Moderate damage	
○ 0 Severe damage	
○ −2 Cortical lysis	

Evaluation zone 2	Evaluation zone 6
○ 4 No damage	No damage 4 ○
○ 2 Moderate damage	Moderate damage 2 ○
○ 0 Severe damage	Severe damage 0 ○
○ −2 Cortical lysis	Cortical lysis −2 ○

Evaluation zones 3	Evaluation zone 5
○ 4 No damage	No damage 4 ○
○ 2 Moderate damage	Moderate damage 2 ○
○ 0 Severe damage	Severe damage 0 ○
○ −2 Cortical lysis	Cortical lysis −2 ○

Total-1 /20 ○ Very good (20–18); ○ Good (16–14); ○ Average (12–10); ○ Poor (<10)
Total-2 /20 ○ Very good (20–18); ○ Good (16–14); ○ Average (12–10); ○ Poor (<10)

Evaluation osseointegration and secondary stability

Evaluation radiolucent line			Osseointegration/secondary stability Types of secondary stability	Raw Sc.	Weighting	Weighted Sc.
Proximal femur (Zones 1, 2 et 6)			1a Global stability 2+	20	0	**20**
1	○ St.1: lucent line absent	10	1b Global stability +	17	+1	**18**
2	○ St.2: lucent line =/<50%	7	1c Proximal stability +	14	0	**14**
3	○ St.3: lucent line >50%	4	2a Proximal stability −	17	−3	**14**
			2b Global stability +/−	14	0	**14**
Distal femur (Zones 3 et 5)			2c Fibrous stability +/−	11	0	**11**
a	○ St.1: lucent line absent	10	3a Diaphyseal stability +	14	−3	**11**
b	○ St.2: lucent line =/<50%	7	3b Distal stability +	11	−3	**8**
c	○ St.3: lucent line >50%	4	3c Fibrous stab.+/Loosening	8	−3	**5**

Osseointegration (raw sc.) **Total** /20 ○ very good (20); ○ good (17); ○ average (14); ○ poor (11–8)
Secondary stab. (weighted sc.) **Total** /20 ○ very good (20–18); ○ good (14); ○ average (11); ○ poor (5–8)

Global radiographic score

Secondary bone stock		Osseointegration/secondary stability
(Total − 2)	——————— + ———————	*(Weighted sc.)*
10 ○ Very good (20–18)	**Global score /20**	10 ○ Very good (20–18)
8 ○ Good (16–14)		8 ○ Good (14)
5 ○ Average (12–10)		5 ○ Average (11)
2 ○ Poor (<10)		2 ○ Poor(5–8)

○ **Very good (20)** ○ **Good(18–16–15)** ○ **Average(13–12)** ○ Poor (=/<10)

Comparative Measurements of the Bone Density

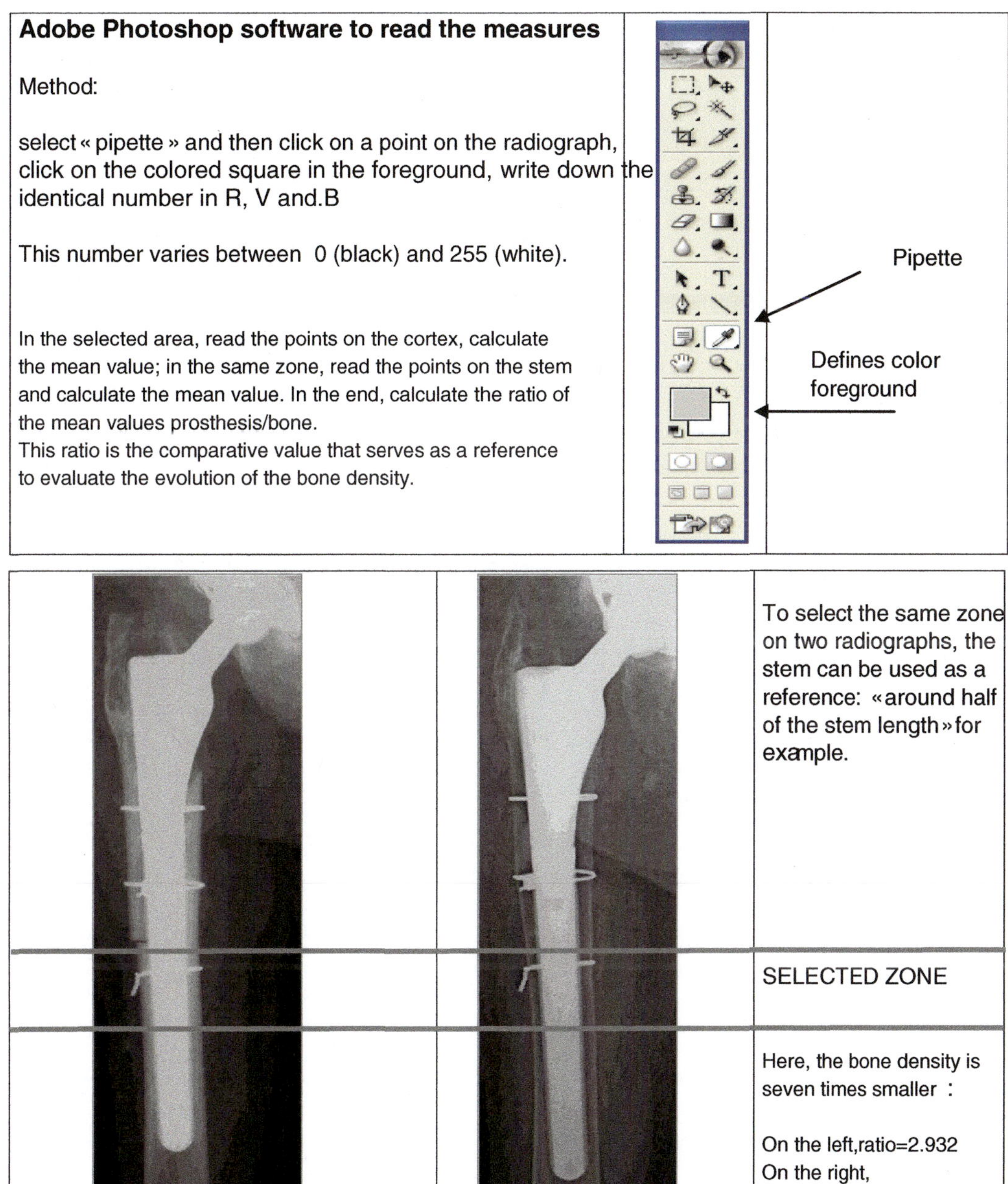

Adobe Photoshop software to read the measures

Method:

select « pipette » and then click on a point on the radiograph, click on the colored square in the foreground, write down the identical number in R, V and.B

This number varies between 0 (black) and 255 (white).

In the selected area, read the points on the cortex, calculate the mean value; in the same zone, read the points on the stem and calculate the mean value. In the end, calculate the ratio of the mean values prosthesis/bone.
This ratio is the comparative value that serves as a reference to evaluate the evolution of the bone density.

To select the same zone on two radiographs, the stem can be used as a reference: «around half of the stem length» for example.

SELECTED ZONE

Here, the bone density is seven times smaller :

On the left,ratio=2.932
On the right, ratio=0.391

Compilation, Transmission, Storage and Update of "Patient" Data

This is a crucial phase without which no reliable study of the results can be made.
- "Patient" data to be collected: clinical and surgical parameters, as well as preoperative and postoperative radiographs.
- Transmission via internet and storage in an officially authorized, secure data base for medical data easily accessible to practitioners and "authorized" services.
1. The collection of the "patient" data is a local application on a PC or iPad.

   It is necessary to have a data capture system that is efficient (i.e. complete), without being plethoric, flexible and simple (i.e. inviting).

Transmission of gathered data should occur in simple and automatic manner.
2. Access to the "patient" data base occurs via internet and can involve several practitioners (or accredited health-care facilities) to ensure sufficient and regular capture of clinical and radiographic data, which is crucial for a reliable evaluation of the results.

- The primary data "suppliers" have to be motivated and dedicated, with the objective, over time, to create a panel of practitioners that becomes a group of experts that can be consulted either before surgery (planning) or after surgery (analysis of the results).

Chapters	Morphotype, Bone defects, Cement, Osteoporosis	
Entrance medical data	**Morphotype**	
Exit medical data	**1- Straight femur in frontal plane** (Slight curvature in sagittal plane)	○ ○
	2- Curved femur in frontal plane (or global curvature in sagittal plane)	○ ○
Preop. clinical condition	**Bone defects** (Isthmus usable)	
Preop. clinical evaluation	**1- No bone defects ou zones 1 and/or 7**	○ ○
Preoperative Rx evaluation	**2- Bone defects zones 2 and/or 6**	○ ○
Operative analysis § implants	**3- Bone defects 1 cort. zones 2-3 or 5-6**	○ ○
	4- Bone defects 2 cort. zones 2-3 and 5-6	○ ○
Analysis of complications	**Cement** (difficulties)	
Postop. immediate Rx eval.	**1- No difficulties**	○ ○
Postoperative clinical eval.	**2- Difficulties**	○ ○
Postop. Rx eval. cup § stem	**Osteoporosis** (IC = épaisseur corticale)	
	1- Very good IC = / > 0,55	○ ○
Eval. Bone stock secondary	**2- Good IC 0,45 - 0,54**	○ ○
Eval. Osseoint./ second. stab.	**3- Average IC 0,35 - 0,44**	○ ○
Global score	**4- Poor IC =/< 0, 34**	○ ○

References

1. Zweymüller KA, Litner FK, Semlitsch MF (1988) Biologic fixation of a press-fit titanium hip joint endoprosthesis. Clin Orthop Relat Res 235:195–199
2. Wagner H (1987) Hip revision prosthesis for cases with severe loss of bone stock [in German]. Orthopade 16:295–300
3. Koster G, Walde TA, Willert HG (2008) Five- to 10-year results using a noncemented modular revision stem without bone grafting. J Arthroplasty 23:964–970
4. Le Béguec P, Sieber HP (2007) Revision of loose femoral prostheses with a stem system based on the "press-fit" principle. Springer, Paris
5. Morscher E (1991) Experience with the press-fit cup and press-fit gliding stem. In: Kusswetter W (ed) Noncemented total hip replacement. International symposium Tubingen, 1990. Inc. Thieme Medical Publishers, New York, pp 221–231
6. Morscher E, Moulin P (1990) Uncemented arthroplasty: Future technology or simple trend? [in French] Communication, Lyon Conference on Hip Surgery
7. Kerboull M (1999) Charnley-Kerboull total hip arthroplasty. Mechanical and technical bases. Long-term results [in French]. Maitr Orthop 83:6–10
8. Blaimont P, Halleux P, Jedwab J (1968) Distribution of load into the femoral bone [in French]. Rev Chir Orthop 54:303–319
9. Essig J, Puget J (1995) 5-year results of a homogeneous series of 74 revision prostheses (PP system). Analysis of the mechanical stability of the implant and bone regeneration [in French]. Rev Chir Orthop 81(Suppl 2):143–144
10. Della Valle CJ, Paprosky WG (2004) The femur in revision total hip arthroplasty evaluation and classification. Clin Orthop Relat Res 420:55–62
11. D'Antonio J, Mc Carthy J, Bargar WL (1993) Classification of abnormalities in total hip arthroplasty. Clin Orthop 296:133–139
12. Vives P, De Lestang M, Pallot R, Cazeneuve JF (1989) Aseptic loosening. Definition-classification [in French]. Rev Chir Orthop 75(Suppl I):29–31
13. Vives P, Picault C (1999) Transfemoral approach and distal locked stem in femoral failures of total hip prosthesis. Sauramps Medical, Montpellier
14. Kerboull M (1996) Treatment of aseptic femoral loosening of total hip prostheses [in French]. Cahiers d'enseignement de la SOFCOT 55:1–17
15. Vielpeau C, Locker B, Van Neverbelde T, Heuguet V (1989) Risk of infection in orthopedic surgery [in French]. Encycl Med Chir Tech Chir 44005:1–18
16. Harris WH (1969) Traumatic arthritis of the hip after dislocation and acetabular fracture. Treatment by Mold arthroplasty. An end-result study using new method of result evaluation. J Bone Joint Surg Am 51:737–754
17. D'Aubigné RM, Postel M (1954) Functional results of hip arthroplasty with acrylic prosthesis. J Bone Joint Surg Am 36A:451–475
18. Engh CA, Massin P, Suthers KE (1990) Roentgenographic assessment of the biologic fixation of porous-surfaced femoral component. Clin Orthop Relat Res 257:107–128
19. Epinette JA, Geesink R, AGORA Group (1994) Proposal of a new system of radiological evaluation of cementless femoral prostheses: ARA score [in French]. Cahiers d'enseignement de la SOFCOT 50:107–120
20. Engh CA, Bobyn JD, Glassman AH (1987) Porous-coated hip replacement. The factors governing bone ingrowth, stress-shielding, and clinical results. J Bone Joint Surg 69B:45–55
21. Boisgard S, Moreau PE, Tixier H, Levai JP (2001) Bone reconstruction, leg length discrepancy, and dislocation rate in 52 Wagner revision total hip arthroplasties at 44-month follow up [in French]. Rev Chir Orthop Reparatrice Appar Mot 87:147–154
22. Tannast M, Zheng G, Anderegg C, Burckhardt K, Langlotz F, Ganz R, Siebenrock KA (2005) Tilt and rotation correction of acetabular version on pelvic radiographs. Clin Orthop Relat Res 438:182–190
23. Shrout PE, Fleiss JL (1979) Intraclass correlations: uses in assessing rater reliability. Psychol Bull 86(2):420–428
24. Gruen TA, McNeice GM, Amstutz HC (1979) "Modes of failure" of cemented stem-type femoral components. A radiographic analysis of loosening. Clin Orthop Relat Res 141:17–27
25. Paprosky WG, Greidanus NV, Antoniou J (1999) Minimum 10-year results of extensively porous-coated stems in revision hip arthroplasty. Clin Orthop Relat Res 369:230–242
26. Abadie P, Lebel B, Pineau V, Burdin G, Vielpeau C (2010) Cemented total hip stem design influence on adaptative cortical thickness and femoral morphology. Orthop Traumatol Surg Res 96(2):104–110
27. Bugbee WD, Culpepper WJ 2nd, Engh CA Jr, Engh CA Sr (1997) Long-term clinical consequences of stress-shielding after total hip arthroplasty without cement. J Bone Joint Surg Am 79:1007–1012
28. Sychterz CJ, Engh CA (1996) The influence of clinical factors on periprosthetic bone remodelling. Clin Orthop Relat Res 322:285–292
29. Kavanagh BF, Fitzgerald RH Jr (1985) Clinical and roentgenographic assessment of total hip arthroplasty. A new hip score. Clin Orthop Relat Res 193:133–140
30. Girard J, Roche O, Wavreille G, Canovas F, Le Béguec P (2011) Stem subsidence after total hip revision: 183 cases at 5.9 years follow-up. Orthop Traumatol Surg Res 97:121–126
31. Korovessis P, Repantis T (2009) High medium-term survival of Zweymüller SLR-plus® stem used in femoral revision. Clin Orthop Relat Res 467(8):2032–2040

9783319036137